KT-574-024

the g.i. diet cookbook

Antony Worrall Thomspon
with Mabel Blades RD & Jane Suthering

Photography by Steve Lee

More than 100 low
glycemic-index recipes for
healthy weight loss

Stewart, Tabori & Chang
New York

To Janet O'Leary, a beautiful lady who has lived with diabetes all her life but hadn't let it get in the way of enjoyment: a true inspiration to me and many others.

Important note

The information and advice contained in this book are intended as a general guide to dieting and healthy eating and are not specific to individuals or their particular circumstances. This book is not intended to replace treatment by a qualified practitioner. Neither the authors nor the publishers can be held responsible for claims arising from the inappropriate use of any dietary regime. Do not attempt self-diagnosis or self-treatment for serious or long-term conditions without consulting a medical professional or qualified practitioner.

Library of Congress Cataloging-in-Publication Data is on file with the Library of Congress.

ISBN: 1-58479-546-8

Text copyright © 2005 by Mabel Blades
Recipes copyright © 2005 by Antony Worrall Thompson, except for Muesli Mix (pg. 46), Apple and Hazelnut Muesli (pg. 46), South African Seed Bread (pg. 52), and Fruited Tea Bread (pg. 54) copyright © 2005 by Jane Suthering
Photography copyright © 2005 by Steve Lee
Book design copyright © 2005 by Kyle Cathie Limited

Published in 2006 by Stewart, Tabori & Chang
An imprint of Harry N. Abrams, Inc.

All rights reserved. No portion of this book may be reproduced, stored in a retrieval system, or transmitted in any form or by any means, mechanical, electronic, photocopying, recording, or otherwise, without written permission from the publisher.

The text of this book was composed in Frutiger and Garamond.

Printed and bound in Singapore
10 9 8 7 6 5 4 3 2 1

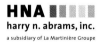

HNA
harry n. abrams, inc.
a subsidiary of La Martinière Groupe

115 West 18th Street
New York, NY 10011
www.hnabooks.com

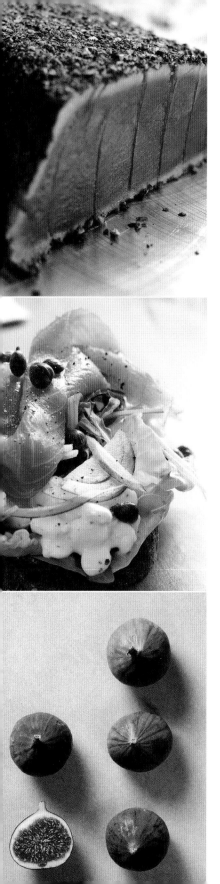

Contents

introduction

So why, I hear you ask, am I writing about a G.I. diet? Simple really, a couple of years ago I was diagnosed with Syndrome X or Metabolic Syndrome (a pre-diabetic state) and I was determined to reverse the situation. This meant a total lifestyle change; I always knew I was overweight, I knew I was unfit but I didn't do anything about it, until I was diagnosed with Syndrome X, that is.

The first step was to get my head around the possibility of becoming diabetic. I looked at all the diabetic cookbooks and thought if that is going to be my food life, then I'm finished! I decided to do some research and realized that it was possible for people with diabetes to have enjoyable food after all, so I wrote *Healthy Eating for Diabetes* in 2003.

From there I wanted to go further in my new healthy eating campaign, especially as obesity is becoming a ticking time-bomb in the UK and other Western countries. I undertook to discover a diet that wouldn't be a fad, but would actually be healthy and help you to lose weight at the same time.

Most diets work in the beginning, but almost all are boring so you tend to veer off the straight and narrow very quickly. But as most diets involve reducing the amount of food you eat, your metabolic rate goes down to compensate for the change, so, as soon as you revert to your normal food regime, your body puts on weight more quickly as it has become used to less food.

What we need is a diet regime with a small "d." A diet that is so enjoyable it can become part of life's routine. Over the last few years our lives have changed beyond recognition—we've become couch potatoes. Gone is exercise, gone are outdoor pursuits, replaced by computer games, remote controls, DVDs, and the like. Similarly with family meals, home cooking has been put on the back burner, we've become content with "ping" cuisine—mediocre ready-made meals packed full of preservatives, salt, sugars, and fats and heated in the microwave. Or we rely on take-out food, which are, for the most part, equally problematic on the health front.

The time has come to review the modern diet. By not enjoying the social stimulation of family get-togethers around the kitchen table, we lose good food, we lose communication skills, we lose the family unit. Too many of us spend our days eating on the run. Proper breakfast has all but disappeared, lunch comes in the form of sugar-based products, after-work drinks are often sugary alcopops, all of which play havoc with blood sugar levels which, in turn, means energy levels fluctuate. So you have an immediate high after lunch, followed by a crash at about 4 p.m. when you feel exhausted. You reach for something sweet, which will only cause your blood sugar levels to shoot up again, only to come crashing down and so the vicious spiral continues.

My G.I. diet deals with these issues, providing exciting dishes for you to enjoy; dishes that will remove the feeling that you are on a diet with a big "D." There is a huge choice of exciting and varied ingredients available to you, and I guarantee that you won't be bored. They are the perfect food for all occasions and, I hope, will give you lots of ideas to generate enthusiasm for a lifestyle change. You will feel better, you will notice improved energy levels, and you can live in the knowledge that you have actually found a diet that is good for you, one that is supported by many top nutritionists. Couple this with a bit more exercise and, hey presto, it's a new you.

You can lead a horse to water, but you can't make it drink: your life, your health is up to you. Good luck.

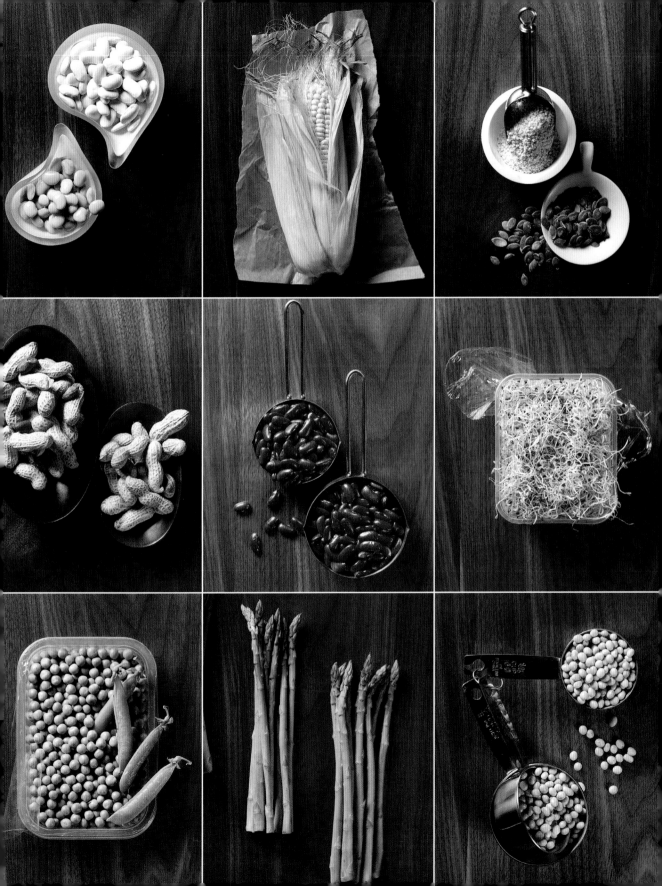

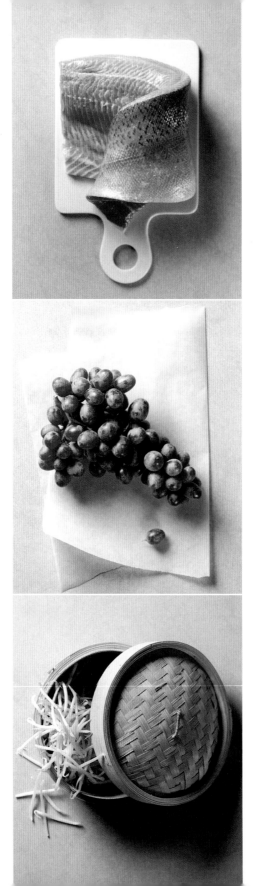

about the g.i.

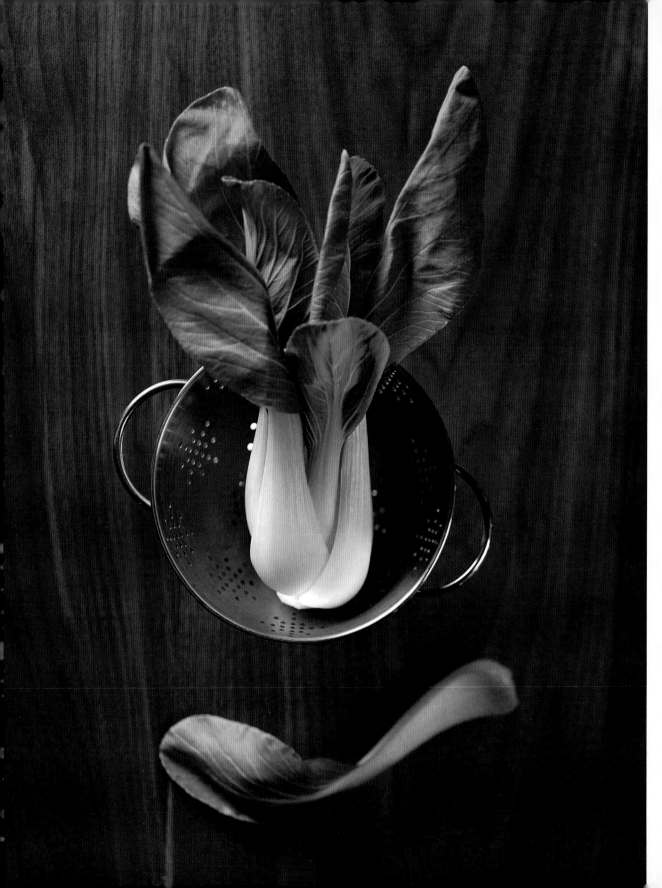

there are no bad foods, just bad diets

What we eat is vital to our health and well-being as well as to how we look, feel, and function. If we do not feel good then we are not getting the most out of life and not doing all those things we really want to do.

As well as achieving good health, it is essential that we also enjoy our food and feel satisfied by it rather than feeling constantly hungry.

This book is about encompassing that principle by eating foods with a low Glycemic Index (G.I.) and low calorie content. Thus it is also about helping people to lose weight and then keep from regaining any weight lost.

Food and dieting

The most important fact to understand is that there are no bad foods, just bad diets with too much fat and sugar and too little fruit and vegetables.

There is nothing wrong with eating a fried breakfast, a cream cake, burger and fries, a bar of chocolate, or a bag of potato chips—provided you only do so occasionally. It is when the whole diet is dominated by these high-fat and high-sugar foods that health problems are likely to occur.

If you divide a plate of food into sections following the recognized guidelines for a balanced diet, there is a place for a small amount of these high-fat and high-sugar foods. So while it is accepted that they provide extra enjoyment and variety to a balanced diet, they should not be eaten to excess.

In the same way, you do not have to concentrate your diet solely on low-G.I. foods, but instead balance your diet by including them where possible. The backbone of this low-G.I. way of eating is about balance, enjoyment, and health.

Unbalanced diets

Unhealthy diets can lead to health problems such as obesity, type 2 diabetes, digestive problems such as irritable bowel syndrome, cancers, and coronary heart disease. Eight guidelines for a healthy diet are:

- Enjoy your food

- Eat a variety of different foods

- Eat the right amount to be a healthy weight

- Eat plenty of foods rich in fiber

- Eat plenty of fruit and vegetables

- Don't eat too many foods that contain a lot of fat

- Don't have sugary foods and drinks too often

- If you drink alcohol, drink sensibly

All these guidelines fit in perfectly with the recipes in this book and will help you to achieve and maintain a sensible weight as well as a nutritionally balanced diet that will help to reduce these health risks.

It matters a great deal that we should take pleasure in our food, purchasing, preparing, and then taking the time to savor the meal. This book is about a way of eating that is not only nutritionally balanced, satisfying, and low in calories, but also delicious. It is not obsessive about calorie counting or indeed about any type of counting: it is just about healthy and enjoyable eating that you can follow for life, without feeling that you are denying yourself certain foods. The guiding principle behind the G.I. diet is that you won't even notice that you are on a diet, thus making it much easier to stick to.

One of the problems with many diets that promote weight loss is that they leave you feeling hungry all the time because the allowed portion sizes of carbohydrates are small. As a result you do not feel satisfied and are tempted by snacks and extra portions of foods.

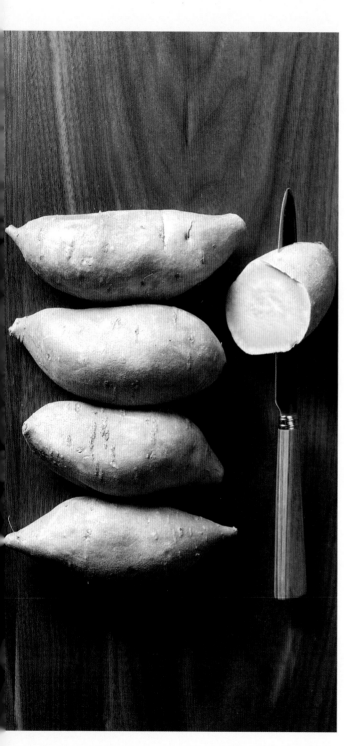

What is different about the G.I. diet?

Simply put, foods with a low G.I. are digested more slowly by the body and this helps to keep the blood sugar at a medium level longer, making us feel satisfied longer and therefore less hungry. Adding these foods to meals will slow the absorption of the whole meal and thus reduce the G.I. of the entire meal. This is a brilliant concept because it means that by adding something to a dish, then you lower the G.I. content of the whole meal.

Meals with a low G.I. are ideal for the whole family as they are easy to incorporate into busy lifestyles as well as family budgets. For children they are particularly satisfying and keep them bursting with energy without continually looking for the next high-fat and high-sugar snack. Meals with a low G.I. are also nutritionally well balanced, which helps to promote growth. Recent research suggests that low-G.I. meals help children to avoid gaining excess weight as the food is so satisfying that they do not want the extra high-calorie snacks. For teenagers who are rushing through life at a hectic pace, they provide all the energy they need and keep the blood sugar at a sustained level longer, which helps them to participate in activities be it sports or dancing the night away.

Foods with a low G.I. are legumes of all types including beans, peas, lentils, whole fruits, oats, grains, bran cereals and multigrain breads, milk and milk products, sweet potatoes, corn and pasta.

Foods with a medium G.I. are pita breads, couscous, boiled potatoes, ice cream, muffins and basmati rice.

Foods with a high G.I. are white and whole-wheat bread and flour, cookies made from them, easy-cook white rice and glucose-based products. These can still be used in dishes provided that they are complemented by ingredients with a low G.I.

what is the glycemic index (g.i.)?

The G.I. is really a measure of how our bodies digest, absorb, and use different carbohydrate foods to provide energy in the body. Carbohydrate foods, or "carbs" as they may be referred to today, are sugars and starches. These should be the main source of energy for our bodies.

Our bodies also derive energy from fat but there is a link between obtaining too much energy from fat (especially saturated fat) and coronary heart disease. High-fat diets can be high in calories, too, and thus contribute to obesity.

Protein foods supply energy to the body as can alcohol, which may account for the fact that a number of overweight men drink a large amount of alcohol.

Types of carbohydrates

During the process of digestion, carbohydrates are broken down into the component simple sugars, or monosaccharides as they are called. The principal one is glucose. This is the tiny molecule that passes through the walls of the intestines and into the bloodstream where it circulates to all the body's cells, which remove the glucose from the blood to provide their energy. Glucose is the main source of energy for all the body's cells.

Sugars other than glucose are called disaccharides and consist of glucose linked with another type of monosaccharide. Sugars such as sucrose, maltose, and lactose are made up of half glucose and half of another type of monosaccharide. Starches are made up of long chains of glucose molecules.

Foods that contain a high proportion of glucose, such as candy, release the glucose rapidly into the bloodstream, while those foods that contain disaccharides and starches take longer as the glucose molecules first have to be released from the food being digested.

Carbohydrate foods include

Sugars of all types such as:

● Sucrose or table sugar, whether white or brown, which is found in a number of foods and drinks. Examples of items that contain large amounts of sugar are cakes, jam, pastries, candies, puddings, chocolates, ice cream, and soft drinks; it is also added to teas, coffees, and cereals.

● Glucose, which is found in sports drinks and used in syrups and food manufacture.

● Fructose, which is found in fresh fruits and juices made from them, as well as processed fruits such as canned and dried fruits, and foods that contain processed fruits such as fruit puddings.

● Lactose, which is the sugar found in milk and milk products such as yogurts.

● Maltose, which is found in malt used for flavorings in cereals.

Starches of all types including those found in foods such as:

● Potatoes, rice, pasta, couscous, noodles, breakfast cereals, crackers, grains of all types such as oats and barley.

● Legumes, which include lentils, dried beans, and dried peas, contain substantial amounts of starchy carbohydrate along with proteins.

Various terms are used for starchy carbohydrates, for example, "unrefined carbohydrates" which refer to those with more fiber such as whole-wheat bread, brown pasta, brown rice, and wholegrain breakfast cereals.

"Refined carbohydrates" are those that have been more highly processed and have had some of the fiber removed; examples include white bread, white pasta, and white rice.

Starchy carbohydrates are considered to be the body's preferred source of energy and it is estimated that they should supply about 45–50 percent of our energy.

Carbohydrates provide 3.75 calories per gram, protein supplies 4 calories per gram, and fat, 9 calories per gram. Alcohol, if we drink it, provides 7 calories per gram. It is therefore clear that a diet high in starchy carbohydrates can be low in calories. Add to this carbohydrates with a low G.I. and you have a really satisfying way of eating.

How food is used in the body

The food we eat provides us with energy for all our activities such as movement, as well as those body functions that we are not aware of, such as maintaining body temperature, providing the energy for body cells, and keeping the heart, lungs, and circulation functioning.

Food also provides us with substances such as proteins, which are needed for the repair and growth of body tissues. Food additionally contains minerals such as calcium, required for the maintenance of bones, and vitamins, necessary to regulate the vast array of processes that occurs in the body.

The process of breaking down the food we eat into tiny molecules that our body can absorb is called digestion. Absorption is the process whereby the tiny molecules of nutrients pass across the wall of the digestive tract and into the bloodstream. These nutrients are then carried around the body in the bloodstream and taken up by those parts of the body that require them. Digestion occurs in the digestive tract, or gut as it is sometimes called. Special substances called digestive enzymes are secreted by various parts of the digestive tract and break down foodstuffs into their component parts.

Digestion and absorption occur mainly in the small intestine, but certain simple substances such as glucose and alcohol are absorbed in the stomach. As a result, glucose enters the bloodstream rapidly, as does alcohol, which is why we start to feel the effects quickly after drinking it.

When the body has to digest carbohydrate foods that have a tougher coat, such as seeds for example, or take longer to break down because of their structure, then their nutrients take longer to enter the bloodstream. If a food is peeled, mashed, or processed before consumption it is easier for the digestive enzymes to attack it and break it down into glucose.

How food affects blood sugar levels

During digestion, sugars and starches are broken down into their component parts of glucose.

When glucose is eaten on its own, it enters the bloodstream rapidly so that the blood glucose level zooms up quickly. The level also falls quickly; indeed it may dip down very rapidly and to a very low level. That is why we often feel hungry again soon after we have eaten a food that causes a rapid rise in blood glucose level because when we have that equally rapid fall, our bodies tell us to eat to boost the blood glucose level up again.

This rise in blood glucose can be measured and this measurement is the basis of the G.I. The level to which the blood glucose rises when a set amount of glucose is taken is given a value of 100. Other foods cause different rises in blood glucose level and thus have a different G.I. (see page 17). Don't worry about these numbers—here the G.I. index is simplified into low, medium, and high G.I. foods.

Foods with a lower G.I. tend to make us feel satisfied for longer and thus less inclined to snack. They are broken down slowly in the digestive tract, producing a slow, steady rise and also a slow fall of the blood glucose level, meaning we have a more even release of energy from the food and we feel less hungry.

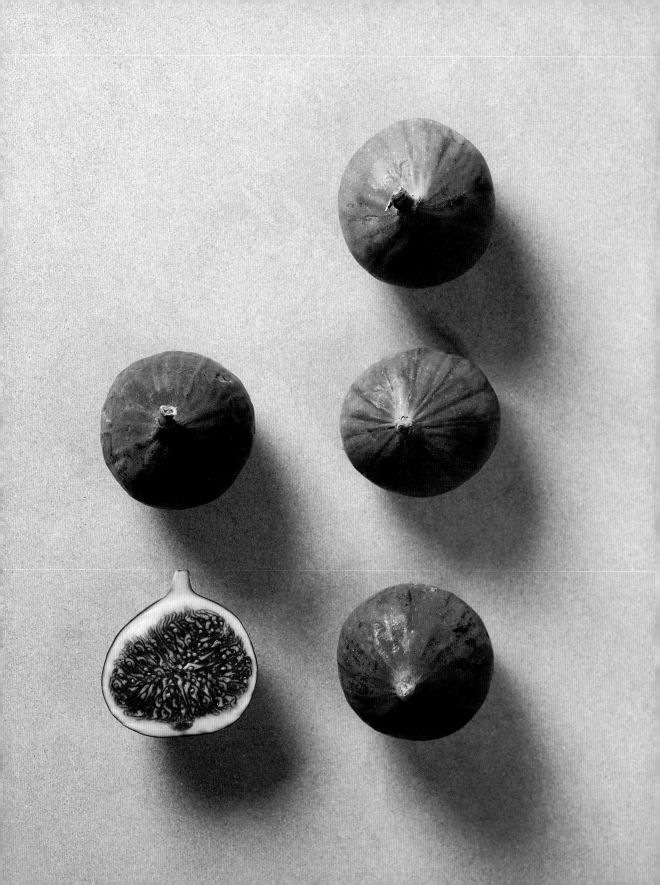

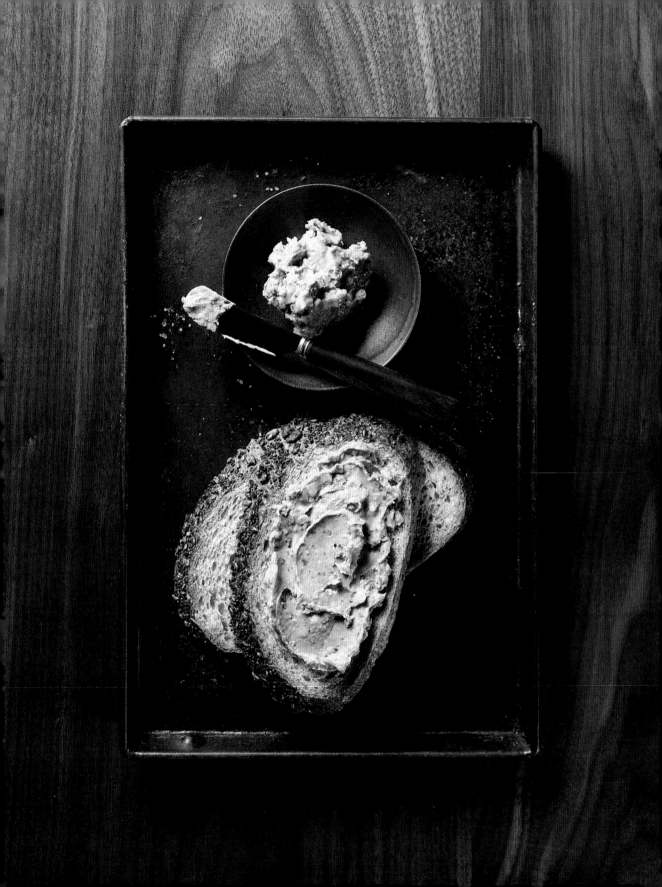

keeping the g.i. low

If you add low-G.I. foods to a meal, they mix with foods with a high G.I. and slow down their digestion and absorption as glucose. So this is a way of eating where you are encouraged to eat more of certain foods.

Many food manufacturers are at present working on studies to find out the different G.I. levels of the foods they make, but it is fairly straightforward to reduce the G.I. of meals by mixing a low-G.I. food with a higher one.

Good examples of this are:

● Serving baked beans in tomato sauce with a baked potato.

● Eating peanut butter on a slice of white toast or whole-wheat toast—it is the peanut butter that reduces the G.I.

● Using grain and seed breads rather than white or brown breads—it is the hard coatings of the seeds and grains that slow down the digestive process and lower the G.I.

● Adding skim milk to breakfast cereals—here it is the skim milk that lowers the G.I.

● Adding extra dried fruit to cake or loaf mixes.

● Having oat biscuits with cheese rather than crackers as the oat biscuits have a lower G.I. than crackers.

● Serving beans or peas which have a low G.I. rather than (or as well as) carrots with a traditional roast.

● Serving more pasta dishes due to the low G.I. of pasta.

● Adding lentils, barley, lima beans, or split peas to your soup to reduce the G.I.

● Making a risotto with basmati rice rather than the traditional arborio rice as it has a lower G.I.

● Having a snack of dried apricots as well as some candies.

what should I count?

Foods with a high G.I. are those with a G.I. above 70, while those with a medium G.I. are in the range 56–69, and those with a low G.I. are 55 or below.

All over the world research projects are being carried out to measure the G.I. of different foods. However, various factors affect these studies, as the rest of the diet and indeed the previous diet and health status of the participants can affect the G.I. And some of the values vary, especially between different brands.

Some researchers suggest using the "Glycemic Loads" of foods rather than the G.I. This is the G.I. multiplied by the amount of carbohydrate in a food. Others have used a G.I. point system, which is a relationship between the G.I. and the energy density of a food.

To achieve weight loss, a calorie reduction is needed and some people therefore advocate counting calories. Counting, listing, and adding up numbers may suit some people but for most it becomes a chore and they soon give up. Sometimes, too, people get it wrong.

So this way of eating is based on the simple principles of a low-G.I. and low-calorie diet.

Portion sizes

The one thing that you should try to keep an eye on is portion size.

To lose weight, the portion sizes should be kept to about 3½ ounces for meats, 3½–5 ounces for fish, 2 ounces for nuts, 1 ounce for cheese, 1–2 eggs per portion at mealtimes and about 2 cups of skim milk per day.

It is boring to be obsessive about portion sizes but try to check their weights on scales or when you buy foods so that you begin to recognize what these foods weigh.

the g.i. food table

Foods with a low G.I.

So which carbohydrate foods have a low G.I.?

Breads, breakfast cereals,
and grains
All-bran
Barley
Buckwheat
Bulgur
Grain breads
Oat bran
Oats
Pasta of all types
Pumpernickel
Rice noodles
Seeded breads
Sourdough rye
Soy and linseed bread
Spelt wheat bread
Toasted muesli
Turkish whole-wheat bread

Vegetables and legumes
Baked beans
Black-eyed peas
Butter beans
Chickpeas
Corn
Kidney beans
Lentils
Lima beans
Navy beans
Peas
Small new potatoes boiled
in skin
Soy beans
Sweet potatoes

Fruits
Apples
Bananas
Cherries
Dried apples
Dried apricots
Grapefruit and its juice
Grapes
Kiwi fruit
Mangoes
Oranges
Peaches
Pears
Plums
Prunes
Strawberries

Snack foods
Apple juice
Cashews
Corn chips
Cranberry juice
Hot chocolate
Grainy fruit loaf
Low-fat chocolate mousse
Low-fat custard
Low-fat yogurt
Malted milk
Minestrone soup
Peanuts
Skim milk
Tomato soup
Tortillas (corn and wheat)

Foods with a medium G.I.

A number of foods are considered to have a medium G.I.

Breads, breakfast cereals,
and cereals
Arborio rice
Arrowroot cookies
Basmati rice
Brown rice
Chapati
Couscous
Crêpes
Croissants
Crumpets
Gnocchi
Hamburger buns
Melba toast
Pita bread
Rice noodles
Rye crispbreads
Whole-wheat rye bread

Vegetables and legumes
Beets
Carrots
Potatoes, peeled and
boiled

Fruits
Canned apricots
Canned fruit cocktail
Canned peaches
Dried figs
Melon
Pineapple

Snack foods
Bean soup
Graham crackers
Quiche
Ice cream
Muesli bars, granola bars
Muffins
Oatmeal cookies
Pea soup
Plain cake
Potato chips
Raisins
Quiche

Foods with a high G.I.

Includes glucose and foods that contain glucose.

Breads, breakfast cereals, and cereals	*Fruits*
Baguettes	Canned lychees
Bagels	Dates
Bread stuffing	Watermelon
Coco Puffs	
Corn Pops	*Snack foods*
Crackers	Doughnuts
Crunchy Nut Cornflakes	French fries—frozen and
Dark rye bread	reheated
Gluten-free bread	Fruit bars
Gluten-free corn pasta	Glucose tablets
Jasmine white rice	Honey
Puffed wheat	Jelly beans
Rice crackers	Morning coffee cookies
Rice Krispies	Plain scones or rolled
Raisin bran	biscuits
Rice	Popcorn
Shredded wheat	Pretzels
Tapioca	Rice cakes
White bread	Glucose-based drinks,
White rice	e.g., sports drinks
Whole-wheat bread	Tofu desserts
	Wafer cookies
Vegetables and Legumes	Waffles
Baked potatoes	
Fava beans	
Mashed potato	
Parsnips	
Pumpkins	
Rutabaga	

Fats, protein, and G.I.

Because fats and protein foods are not made up of glucose units, it means that they all have a G.I. of 0. Adding a low-G.I. food to meals can reduce the overall G.I. of the meal as it mixes with the other foods and slows down digestion and absorption.

This means that adding oils, fats, and cream to dishes reduces the G.I. of a meal. However, adding more fat to meals means that their calorie value shoots up and if too many calories are eaten then weight is gained rather than lost.

Nonetheless the concept of adding something to meals to reduce the G.I. can be promoted: using small amounts of fats and oils for cooking and for spreading on bread can be helpful as well as adding extra flavor.

Other foods such as those that supply protein not only balance a meal from a nutritional point of view but also reduce the G.I. Therefore eating these foods as part of a meal will actually reduce the G.I. (but note portion sizes—see page 17):

● Skim milk or low-fat milk, which has a low-G.I. value because it contains the milk sugar lactose

● Eggs

● Very low-fat cheeses

● Low-fat yogurts

● Lean meats such as beef, pork, and lamb as well as their livers and kidneys

● Poultry such as chicken and turkey without skin

● Game such as hare, rabbit, pigeon, and pheasant

● Fish and shellfish of all types

● Nuts of all types and nut spreads such as peanut butter

how the g.i. can help

Diabetes

Diabetes is a common disorder whereby the body does not produce enough insulin or produces ineffective insulin, which the body needs to enable all its cells to take up glucose. There are two types of diabetes:

Type 1 where the pancreas stops producing insulin: this type of diabetes affects mainly children and younger people. It usually has a rapid onset with severe symptoms such as weight loss; excessive thirst, and even coma can develop. This type of diabetes needs insulin for treatment.

Type 2 which mainly affects older people and those who are overweight. The onset is often very slow and many people are found to have type 2 diabetes after having a routine medical or even an eye test. The symptoms tend to vary and be less acute than those for type 1 diabetes. Symptoms include thirst, passing urine frequently, and tiredness.

Whichever the type of diabetes, the blood glucose level rises above the normal level as the production of insulin is not working properly. Altering the diet to maintain a lower blood glucose level is therefore fundamental to control the condition.

Thus an eating pattern where low-G.I. foods are included enables the blood sugar level to be well controlled and assists in the long-term management of diabetes. Many of those with type 2 diabetes are overweight, so eating a low-calorie, low-G.I. diet is excellent for promoting weight loss and hence long-term control of the diabetes.

Good control of the blood glucose level means that diabetes sufferers have a reduced risk of developing any of the complications associated with the condition.

Syndrome X

This is considered to be a metabolic disorder that could lead to future heart problems, type 2 diabetes, strokes, and diseases that affect the blood vessels and circulation. At present it is thought that this condition is very common and probably affects a quarter of those over 20 years of age and half of those over 50.

Syndrome X is associated with abdominal fat deposition which results in a waist that is nearly as large or larger than the hips giving the so-called apple shape (see also page 24). It is also linked with low levels of the protective cholesterol in the blood and high levels of another sticky substance called triglycerides circulating in the blood. Also insulin resistance, where the insulin does not work correctly, occurs, which causes raised levels of blood glucose. High blood pressure levels are also found.

Doctors or nurses can offer tests for all these factors. However, a diet rich in low-G.I. foods will help to maintain low blood sugar levels, while a low-calorie diet for weight loss will help to control Syndrome X.

Digestive disorders and IBS

Many people suffer from digestive and bowel problems such as irritable bowel syndrome (IBS). Eating adequate amounts of foods that are slowly digested, and which also contain fiber and are low in fat, accompanied by drinking adequate amounts of fluid greatly assists those with bowel problems such as IBS.

Foods with a low G.I. are beneficial in promoting a healthy flora of bacteria in the bowel and intestines, which reduces bloating, bowel disorders, and also food sensitivities.

Other health problems helped by low-G.I. meals

A number of other health problems are helped by a diet with a low G.I. Such disorders include:

Polycystic ovary syndrome where the maintenance of the blood glucose level can help to control symptoms and aid weight loss.

Coronary heart disease and raised lipid levels in the blood are assisted by a diet that maintains the blood sugar level without the peaks and troughs found in a diet with high-G.I. foods. This diet is also low in fats and therefore helps to prevent coronary heart disease.

Hypoglycemia, with the repeated low blood sugar level and symptoms of shakiness that occur, is helped by the maintenance of the blood sugar level which results when a low-G.I. diet is followed.

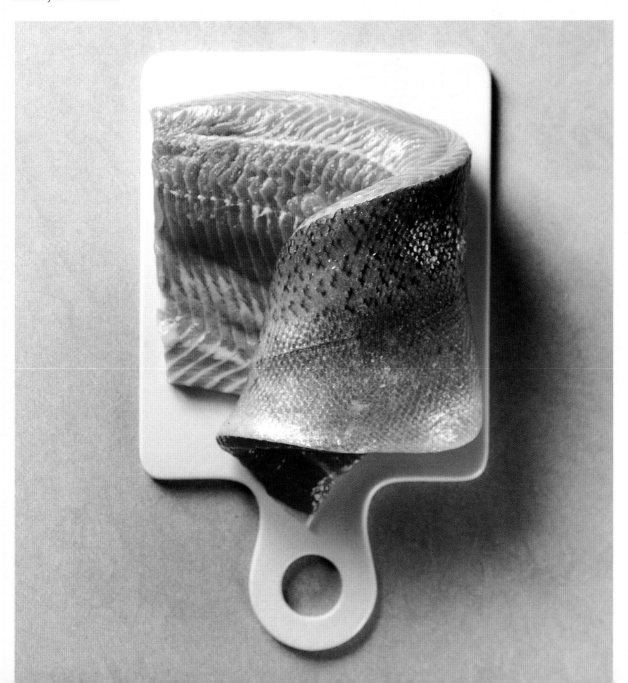

weight loss and the g.i.

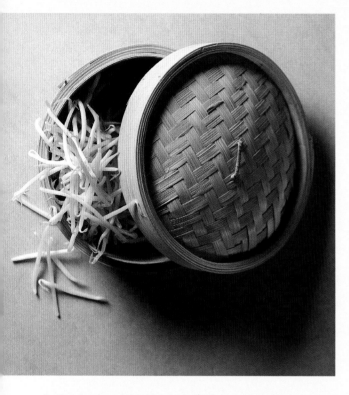

In the developed world, over half of the population is overweight or obese. Many people are concerned about their weight and move from one sort of diet to another, which means they veer from one type of eating to another with the consequence that weight is lost and then regained, often with even more gained besides.

This book will help those who are overweight to lose weight by following a diet that is low in G.I. as well as low in calories. It enables readers to reduce the G.I. level of their foods and thus helps them to feel more satisfied after eating. The recipes are inspirational and give a tempting array of calorie-counted dishes (as well as being low in fat and salt) that can be included in a low-calorie diet to bring about sensible weight loss that can be maintained.

This way of eating thus becomes enjoyable and can be maintained not just for weeks or months, but long-term.

As the concept of G.I. is fairly new, there are few studies on it, but those there are show that it is helpful in promoting a slow, steady weight loss with no hunger pangs.

Long-term weight loss

There is no point in losing weight just to put it back on again. Indeed it is unhealthy for your weight to yo-yo up and down.

All too often people regard diets as short term. This one is not a diet for a short time but an improved way of eating that can be sustained for life and in all situations, so that any weight lost remains lost!

This way of eating has no forbidden foods, just a healthy diet with extras of low-G.I. foods to sustain a healthy blood sugar level.

Being overweight

The weight that anyone who is overweight needs to lose is fat. Most people would love to lose it quickly and indeed at many slimming groups those who lose the most weight each week are applauded and rapid weight loss is celebrated.

A rapid weight loss may well be due to a loss of fluid and muscle as well as fat. This is likely to result from a strict diet, which means there is no education in eating habits. So when the diet is given up, any weight lost returns—and usually with a bit extra. If muscle tissue is lost then it is often replaced with more fat, which is an unhealthy type of tissue.

Quite honestly, as a dietitian dealing with someone who has been overweight for a long time, my goal is first to stop the person continuing to gain weight and then to maintain their weight for a few weeks. This gives them confidence not only for a long-term weight loss but also for maintaining a new, low weight when that is achieved. Next I encourage a slow, steady weight loss of 1–2¼ pounds per week. This means that body fat is being shed and also the person is gradually adjusting their diet into their ordinary lifestyle, making it easier to keep to the new eating pattern.

Not only can they keep to the new eating pattern but they can also enjoy feeling full, and fit the major principles of the new way of eating into family meals, eating out, parties, and the general rush of 21st-century living.

How it happens

The basic reason why people become overweight is that they consume too many calories from food for their own individual needs. They then store these calories up as fat both under the skin and around the vital organs.

It is so easy to be tempted to eat more than we need with the readily available range of foods everywhere we go. In an age when everyone is extremely busy with work, home life, and traveling to and from places, it is difficult to find enough time to buy and prepare meals. Also, many people are unsure about what to buy for a well-balanced diet and how to cook various foods. Thus any hunger pangs are easily satisfied by grabbing a quick snack on the way to work, another from the snack cart at mid-morning, a fast-food lunch fitted in between shopping, chocolate and potato chips bought on the way home at the gas station, a quick and easy microwave dinner containing few vegetables, and then snacks in the evening between chores. All the time we are snacking on these highly processed foods our blood glucose level will be bouncing up and down, making us feel continually hungry and continuing the cycle.

Constantly eating high-calorie snacks means we keep up the vicious cycle of piling on weight because it becomes more difficult to make the effort involved to eat properly.

Problems associated with being overweight
As anyone who is overweight knows, there are a number of issues that have to be faced on an everyday basis. These include the sinking feeling when clothes do not fit anymore and we feel that we are not as healthy as we once were. Stairs become more of an issue as rushing up them causes breathlessness, so we take the elevator and therefore expend fewer calories. People who are overweight may also feel self-conscious about their bodies and so may be less inclined to undertake any sport or activity that demands revealing clothing such as a swimsuit or shorts and as a result undertake less exercise.

They are also less likely to have self-confidence: many overweight people are locked into a cycle of poor self-esteem which affects their relationships, career, activities, and how they look after themselves—for example, many will not spend much on their appearance and plan to do so only when they have lost weight. Many of my really obese patients are almost housebound because of their sheer bulk.

There are obviously many health problems associated with being overweight and these include:

- Coronary heart disease

- Type 2 diabetes

- Joint problems such as arthritis and back problems

- Certain types of cancers

- High blood pressure

- Slower recovery from surgery

- Depression

- Fertility problems

- Gallstones

- Breathing difficulties

How "overweight" is measured

There are various ways of measuring obesity. The ones commonly seen are the height/weight charts, which show a relationship between weight and height and suggest ideal weights.

More recently Body Mass Indexes (BMIs) have been used, which are a more complex relationship between height and weight. To work out your BMI, take your weight in kilograms (2.2 pounds) and divide it by the square of your height, measured in meters (39.4 inches) (BMI = weight in kg ÷ height in metres^2). Fortunately there are charts that show BMIs and make individual calculations unnecessary. The BMIs are categorized into various levels, which show the associated health risks:

A BMI below 20 signifies someone being underweight.

A BMI between 20 and 25 is the normal weight range at which there are few health risks.

A BMI between 26 and 30 signifies the range where someone is regarded as being overweight.

A BMI between 30 and 40 is the range regarded as obese and associated with numerous health risks.

A BMI above 40 signifies someone being severely obese and is strongly associated with health problems.

Often moving from one BMI category to a lower one motivates people to lose weight and thus reduce their health risks.

The worst place for anyone to have fat deposited is around the waist and middle area—the so-called apple shape, as opposed to the pear shape, where weight is deposited around the hips.

A good and effective measure of overweight and obesity is therefore to measure the waist. Generally men should have a waist measurement of below 37 inches and women a measurement of below 31 inches. This is quick and easy to do and needs only a tape measure.

Calorie content of meals

Calories are the units for the measurement of energy and apply both to the energy content of foods as well as that energy expended in activities.

In general, an adult man needs about 2,500 calories per day and a woman 2,000 calories. To lose weight we need to take in fewer calories than we expend so that the fat stores in the body are burned up for our energy needs.

Reducing calorie intake
It is best to make only small adjustments initially and try to keep to around 1,500 calories per day for women wanting to lose weight and 2,000 calories per day for men.

A pound of fat contains about 3,500 calories, so to lose this amount of weight in a week, a reduction of 3,500 calories is needed. Therefore, if the calorie content of a diet is adjusted down by about 500 calories per day, this level of weight loss will be achieved.

Keep to this reduction of about 500 calories per day and at the same time increase exercise levels. As you become fitter it is easy to increase the amount of exercise taken. Thus weight loss is continued. Only reduce the amount of calories further if you have not lost any weight for three to four weeks.

Such a reduction is actually quite easy to do, as only small adjustments have to be made to your diet, such as reducing the amount of spreads put on bread, swapping some of the high-fat and high-sugar snacks for fruit and snacks with a low G.I., avoiding fried foods and high-fat items such as creamy sauces and pastries. Introducing Antony's recipes into your diet will ensure your meals are low in G.I. and calories.

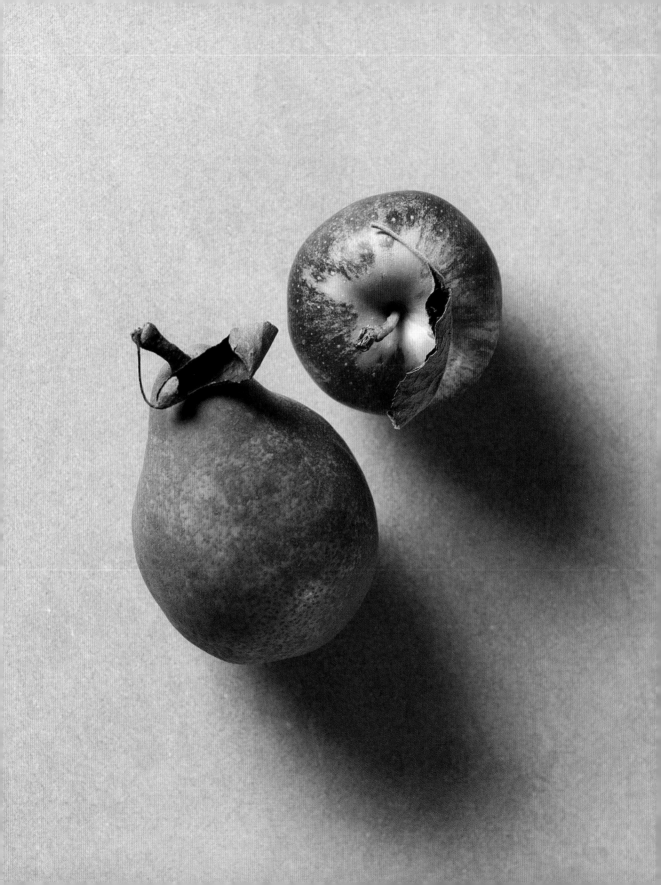

The recipes in this book are all below 300 calories per portion when weight loss is wanted and below 500 calories where weight maintenance is desired (marked by a green semicircle with +300 inside meaning it contains more than 300 calories).

While it can be tedious for some people to write down everything they eat, others find it helpful—so do which you prefer. However, one invaluable tip is to plan a week's menus based on ideas and recipes from this book so that you have something to look forward to and can plan shopping trips for ingredients accordingly.

If you have a period when you find reducing the calorie level difficult, for example over the Christmas season, do not get disheartened, just go back to the main principles of the diet as soon as life permits.

Exercise

Exercise strengthens the muscles including the heart, which is after all, just a muscle, and thus some type of exercise needs to be taken to promote weight loss. Exercise results in an increase in energy expenditure that will help to burn up calories and achieve a greater weight loss than the 500-calorie reduction each day alone. This means that diet is not your only means of losing weight.

Our lifestyle today tends to reduce daily activity levels and it is the little things that add up to make a difference to them. Think of the inventions that have caused a reduction in daily energy expenditure today: using down comforters rather than walking around the bed to tuck in sheets and blankets; using clothes dryers rather than hanging out the wash; using remote controls instead of getting up to switch channels; and using suitcases with wheels rather than having to carry them.

To try to increase exercise levels on a daily basis initially means making several small changes: use the stairs; get up and stand when answering the phone; walk rather than drive; get off the bus one stop early. Most effective is to walk more and do more regular exercise.

Ideally, you should do 30 minutes of exercise each day, sustained for at least 10 minutes at a time. Going to a gym, taking classes for different exercises, dancing, playing team sports, and swimming are all excellent, but many people find that with a busy lifestyle they do not have time to fit such activities into their schedule.

Walking is therefore an ideal exercise that most people can incorporate into their day. I find two ways helpful to encourage walking:

First, I often urge people to buy a pedometer and to wear it to measure the number of steps they take in a day. Some of the more inactive people only take about 1,500 but they then try to improve on their own levels by taking 1,510 the next day and so on until they reach the recommended 10,000 steps per day.

The second way that I encourage people to walk is to ask them to go out of their door and walk for five minutes and then to turn around and try to get home in less than five minutes. This is such a quick and easy way of doing extra walking that many find it fun and take children and partners with them.

Stress and relaxation

When they are stressed, some people "comfort eat" and are less likely to motivate themselves into doing exercise. Therefore it is important for everyone to include some time for relaxation in their schedule. This relaxation may be achieved in many ways, even by exercise or going for a walk. Often just getting outside into the fresh air is in itself relaxing.

Other forms of relaxation can be formalized using relaxation techniques of clearing the mind and slowing down breathing rates; or they can be something as simple as browsing around the stores, stroking the cat, reading, listening to music, or even playing with the children.

nutrition

This is an absolutely fascinating subject with research appearing all the time with new information about the actions of foods in the body as well as different substances found in foods. The whole area of G.I. is relatively new but one that is based on good scientific analysis of foods.

Unfortunately, nutrition abounds with various terms and abbreviations, which are often irrelevant to everyday eating. People put foods together as meals, and factors other than nutritional content come into play when eating.

The concept of the G.I. and low-calorie foods can be based on straightforward principles about foods and suggestions of different combinations of foods to eat rather than on complex calculations. This means that the diet can be easily adopted and become a long-term way of eating which encompasses all the realities of life such as vacations and meals out.

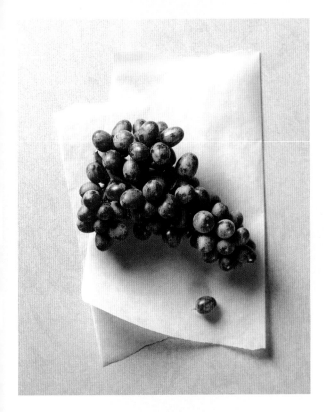

Energy

All foods provide us with energy and eating too much of any of them can make us gain weight. However, if foods are really satisfying, such as those carbohydrates with a low G.I., it is difficult to eat very large amounts of them.

As already mentioned, energy is measured in calories, the term most commonly known, or kilocalories; the metric measurement is joules.

Carbohydrates are the least concentrated source of energy so they are excellent for filling up on. Fats, and foods containing them in quantity, are a more dense energy source than carbohydrates and can also be easily eaten in large amounts, thus forming the basis of a high-calorie diet. Alcohol must be taken into account in the overall calorie intake and failure to do so may well lead to weight gain.

Some carbohydrate foods such as sugars supply "empty calories," which means that they do not supply any nutrients other than calories.

Carbohydrate and fiber

Carbohydrate foods with a low G.I. are those that are slowly broken down into the component glucose molecules, which are then absorbed. If the carbohydrates are associated with dietary fiber, such as skins, pips and seeds, then this slows down the digestive process and their absorption.

Dietary fiber used to be called roughage but is now correctly called non-starch polysaccharide or NSP. Too little dietary fiber is linked with a number of health problems including diverticular disease, bowel cancer, and constipation. We are advised to eat about ¾ ounce of dietary fiber each day but on average we eat just over ½ ounce, so it is little surprise that we see an increase in these problems.

The two types of dietary fiber

The first is soluble fiber, which is smooth and viscous and is found in foods such as oats, barley, and dried legumes (peas, beans, and lentils) as well as in fruit and vegetables. This type of fiber is associated with slowing down digestion in the small intestine and moderating blood sugar and blood cholesterol levels. This is the fiber found in many foods with a low G.I., which is why they have beneficial effects on the blood glucose level.

The second type is insoluble fiber which adds bulk in the bowel by holding onto water and this is the type associated with bran, whole-wheat cereals, whole-wheat flour, brown pasta, and brown rice.

Both types of fiber are valuable but the soluble fiber, and thus many of the carbohydrate foods with a low G.I., is particularly useful for those with diabetes and raised cholesterol levels.

Fruit and vegetables

It is recommended that we all eat five portions of fruit and vegetables per day. (That is fruit and vegetables combined, not five portions of each.) However if we can manage more than the five portions, that is really good news, as most fruit and vegetables have a low G.I.

These five portions are based on the World Health Organization's recommendation that we should eat 14 ounces of fruit and vegetables each day for the health benefits they provide.

The term fruit and vegetables includes all types with the exception of potatoes, which are considered to be a starchy carbohydrate food, as are plantains or green bananas.

It should also be noted that as leafy green vegetables such as lettuce, cabbage, broccoli, and Brussel sprouts all contain little carbohydrate, they have a negligible G.I.

So what is a portion of fruit or vegetables?

Half a large fruit such as a grapefruit.

One medium-sized fruit such as a medium apple, pear, banana, or peach.

One teacup of small fruits such as cherries, Damson plums, or grapes.

A slice of melon, pineapple, or mango—each 1 inch wide.

Two small fruits such as plums.

One tablespoon of dates or dried apricots or raisins or one of the small matchbox-size packs of dried fruits.

Three tablespoons of canned or stewed fruit.

Two tablespoons of cooked, frozen, or canned vegetables. This equates to 3 ounces of vegetables. If this is a dried legume vegetable such as peas, beans, or lentils it only counts as one portion no matter how much is eaten in a day.

A bowl of salad.

A small glass or carton of fruit juice. Fruit juice counts as only one portion no matter how much is drunk in a day.

Many fruits such as grapefruit, cherries, mangoes, oranges, peaches, pears, grapes, and plums have a low G.I., as can be seen from the list on page 18, and are therefore a valuable addition to meals. A further plus is that fruit is low in calories.

But even fruit with a relatively high G.I., such as melon, is low in calories and useful to add to any diet. Dates, despite their high G.I., can be used for sweetening and are much more beneficial than white sugar.

Fruit is a source of vitamins that act as powerful antioxidants, which have a protective effect on the immune system of the body and are associated with lower levels of cancers and coronary heart disease.

To keep the G.I. value of fruit and vegetables as low as possible, eat them unpeeled and cook in chunks rather than mashing or pureeing them. In this way, the digestive process has to work harder and the G.I. level is lowered.

Dairy foods

Dairy foods such as milk and yogurt and foods made from milk such as milkshakes and custards are all excellent sources of calcium in the diet. Because milk contains the sugar lactose, they also have a low G.I. value. These foods are relatively low in calories and can be used to advantage in reducing the G.I. while adding that all-important source of calcium.

Calcium is important for bone health and we need a regular intake. Other sources are hard cheeses, which have a G.I. of 0 but which are relatively high in calories due to the fat content. Fish with bones are another source of calcium.

To keep the calorie level of the diet low choose skim milk, low-fat cheeses such as Edam, or use only small portions of full-fat cheeses. Eat diet yogurts and low-fat *fromage frais* to keep the calorie level down. For those who drink soy milk or rice milk it is important to choose one with added calcium.

Whole milk contains at least 3.5 percent fat, low-fat milk .5 to 2 percent fat, and skim or nonfat milk less than .5 percent fat. Children up to the age of 2 should be given whole milk and low-fat (or 1% or 2%) milk can be introduced thereafter. Skim milk can be given to children from 5 years of age.

Vegetarian and vegan diets

Anyone following a vegetarian or vegan diet often has a head-start in reducing the G.I. of their meals as they tend to use more low-G.I. foods such as dried legumes, nuts, and seeds.

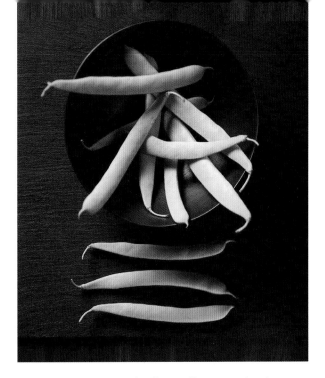

For vegetarians, eggs and milk as well as vegetarian cheese can be included, which will provide protein. Meat is a major source of iron so excluding it means that an alternative source such as dried legumes or nuts or products made from them should be eaten. The iron in meat is in the heme form, similar to the hemoglobin that circulates in our blood, so it is well absorbed, while that from plant sources is in the non-heme form and is poorly absorbed. Vitamin C, which is found in fruit and vegetables, aids the absorption of non-heme iron.

Fats

There are various types of fats but whether saturated, polyunsaturated, or monounsaturated, all fats provide 9 calories per gram and are thus equal as a source of energy. Too much energy in the diet can contribute to weight gain and for health it is recommended that we should obtain no more than 35 percent of energy from the fat in the diet.

Although fats have a G.I. of 0 and can therefore reduce the overall G.I. of a meal or dish, adding fat is not a good way of manipulating the G.I. as it adds extra unwanted calories.

Saturated fats
These are derived from animal sources such as whole milk and cheese, lard, butter, coconut cream, the fat found on

meat and other fatty foods such as pastry dough. They are less desirable because they have been linked with coronary heart disease.

Polyunsaturated fats
Polyunsaturated fats are derived from plant oils such as soybean and corn. These oils are thought to be beneficial, particularly to heart health, but still provide a source of calories.

Essential fatty acids
Omega-3 fatty acids can help prevent blood clotting so they are particularly helpful in preventing coronary heart disease. They are also helpful in preventing inflammation and thus may be beneficial in joint diseases. Sources of omega-3 fatty acids are fish oils, particularly those from oily fish such as salmon, trout, pilchards (large sardines), mackerel, and sardines.

These special fatty acids are also found in linseeds and soybeans—both of which have a low G.I. and are perfect for adding to salads and casseroles.

Omega-6 fatty acids can help prevent coronary heart disease as they reduce levels of the harmful LDL cholesterol. Sources of omega-6 fatty acids are sunflower oil, corn oil, and soybean oils.

Monounsaturated fats
Monounsaturated fats are found in olive oil and rapeseed oil (canola or lear oil) and are considered to be beneficial to the heart.

Trans fats
Most natural fats contain cis bonds. This cis bond is the way in which the chemical elements in the fatty acids are joined together. However, in manufacturing margarines and shortenings, which are used in manufacturing cookies and cakes, the polyunsaturated fats are hydrogenated and more trans fatty acid bonds are formed as the cis bonds are broken and reformed in the trans form.

These trans fatty acids are considered to be similar to saturated fats in their effect on health and are linked with coronary heart disease.

Cholesterol
This is a sticky wax-like substance. It is vital for life and is involved in making essential substances in the body such as cell membranes and hormones. Cholesterol circulates in the blood in two forms and can indicate a risk of coronary heart disease. There are two types of cholesterol:

Low density lipoprotein cholesterol (LDL): the more harmful type of cholesterol.

High density lipoprotein cholesterol (HDL): the beneficial type of cholesterol.

A high proportion of saturated fat in the diet predisposes the production of the more harmful type of cholesterol. Some foods such as liver, egg yolks, and shellfish are naturally a source of cholesterol. There is no need for most people to avoid these nutritious foods but anyone who has high levels of the harmful type of cholesterol may have been advised to limit their consumption of them.

Fluid

Fluid is absolutely essential to health and it is important to drink enough fluid each day. Ideally we should drink 8 cups or glasses of fluid each day. The preferred fluid to rehydrate the body is water.

About 70 percent of the body is fluid and all the vital actions that occur in the body take place in a liquid environment. Adequate fluid is especially needed for the digestive processes to function properly. A lack of fluid can result in numerous problems including tiredness and irritability.

Sometimes it seems to me when dealing with overweight people that they think they are hungry and eat rather than recognize the body's signals of thirst. The amount of fluid they consume is very low but the number of snacks is disproportionately very high. Thus they never feel properly satisfied. In some individuals, just getting them to drink more seems to curtail their appetite for snacks.

Teas, coffees, and colas are useful to add variety but most are a source of caffeine, which acts as a diuretic and makes the body lose fluid. Avoid adding sugar to drinks and also choose low-calorie or sugar-free drinks rather than those that contain sugar, which will add extra calories.

Fruit juices are relatively high in calories and are best diluted with water. Sugary drinks also have a high G.I.

Alcohol

Alcohol can provide a pleasant and relaxing extra to many people's daily intake. There is nothing wrong with this; indeed, a little alcohol, especially red wine, each day is considered to be beneficial to heart health.

As regards health, alcohol is measured in units with 1 unit of alcohol being equivalent to a 4-ounce glass of wine, shot of spirits, 10 ounces of beer, or alcoholic cider, and a small 3-ounce schooner of sherry. Many of the stronger beers and alcohol-based mixer drinks contain 2 or more units per serving.

The British government recommendations as regards alcohol are for women to have not more than 21 units per week and for men not more than 28 units per week. This does not mean that you can save up the whole week's units and take them as a binge one single evening as this can have disastrous effects on health.

As regards calories in alcohol, 10 ounces of beer provides about 90–120 calories, a small glass (about 3 ounces) of wine about 70 calories, and some of the "alcopop" and mixed drinks between 150 and 200 calories per bottle, so the calories soon add up. Try to ensure any mixers are of the low-calorie type. Also have a glass of water for every glass of alcohol taken, to limit the intake and also reduce the adverse effects that alcohol has on hydration.

Excess alcohol is linked with liver cirrhosis and provides extra calories. It is recommended that we all have an alcohol-free day per week to allow the liver cells to regenerate.

Salt

At present we consume an average of 9–12g (1¾-2½ tsps) of salt per person per day when we actually only need about 6g (1¼). Salt is made up of sodium and chloride with about 1g of sodium in 2.5g of salt. Sodium has a harmful effect on blood pressure. Six grams (1¼ tsp) of salt contains about 2.5g of sodium.

Salt is particularly found in manufactured foods such as canned soups, canned vegetables and meals; it is also found in savory snacks such as potato chips and salted peanuts. Foods such as cheese, bacon and ham, and salted fish contain salt, where it is used as a preservative. Sodium is also found in monosodium glutamate, which is used as a flavor-enhancer in manufactured foods such as ready-made meals.

Fresh food such as fruit and vegetables as well as meat, milk, and eggs are all low in sodium. It is best to use a minimum of salt, and gradually reducing the amount of salt in both cooking and sprinkled on food can allow the taste buds to change and become accustomed to less salt.

In general, the recipes in this book contain a low level of salt, i.e., below 0.5g per portion. However, ingredients such as cheese, shellfish, bacon, ham, canned vegetables, soy sauce, blood sausages and other sausages, and fish sauce all contain salt which is required for their preservation and production. Therefore recipes containing these ingredients will have a higher level of sodium. Choose low sodium options such as light soy sauce, low-salt stock cubes, and beans canned in water where possible.

Although it is important to keep salt levels low, remember that this is a salt intake averaged over a period of days so the odd higher salt recipe can be balanced out by a low salt one.

Vitamins and mineral supplements

These are the micronutrients that are needed in tiny amounts—some as little as millionths of a gram—but which are essential to keep us healthy. If we eat a wide variety of foods then we are likely to get everything we need in our diet.

food labeling

A low-G.I. diet focuses on lots of fresh and simple foods and thus contains a range of vitamins and minerals. However, with rushed and skipped meals as well as an occasional prevalence of highly processed foods, we may not get as well balanced an intake of vitamins as we should.

Some groups, such as women who wish to become pregnant or who are in the early stages of pregnancy, are recommended to take a supplement of folic acid.

For those who follow a vegan way of eating, their diet can be low in iron or vitamin B_{12} (meat is a major source of iron, and vitamin B_{12} is found in foods such as meat, fish, milk, and eggs). Vitamin B_{12} is also found in yeast products and if these are not eaten, then vegans may need a supplement.

People following a milk-free diet may be at risk of not taking enough calcium, and supplements can be useful here. For other people, a multi-vitamin and mineral supplement may be beneficial each day if their diet is erratic at times.

The manufacturers of processed foods are required by law to list the ingredients they contain in descending order of quantity. Reading a food label can produce a few surprises when you find that the fish pie contains sugar and the can of carrots, an amount of salt and coloring.

Many labels provide nutritional information and now some food labels are giving information on the G.I. This usually indicates that a food has a low, medium, or high G.I. content.

Food labels contain information on food additives and these items are usually towards the bottom of the list of ingredients as they tend to be present in tiny amounts. Without the use of additives and food preservation techniques, we could not easily have our present lifestyle, but we should try to minimize our intake.

By following a low-G.I. diet and eating more fruit and vegetables—which are fresh and therefore unlabeled—you will soon reduce the overall level of additives in the diet.

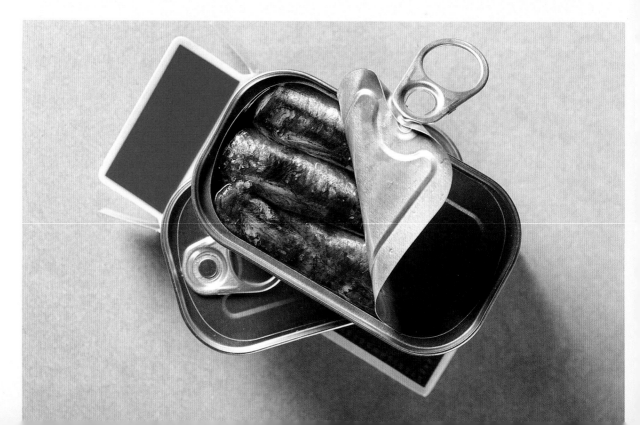

low g.i. tips

Low-G.I. meals

To follow this way of eating there is no need to be obsessive: just try to reduce the G.I. content of some of the carbohydrate foods you eat.

Suggestions for Main meals

Curries made with chickpeas and lentils

Pasta dishes served with sauces containing meat or beans and lots of vegetables and tomatoes instead of cream

Stir-fries with lots of vegetables, beans, and peas

Use basmati rice

Use beans in as many dishes as possible, such as chilies

Suggestions for Dessert

Chunky fruit salads

Compôtes made with dried fruits

Crumbles that include oats

Fresh fruits

Ice cream and fruits

Milk puddings

How to reduce the G.I. content of a day's menu

There are quite a few easy changes you can make to reduce the G.I. of a day's menu.

Breakfast can include oatmeal, grapefruit, a low-G.I. cereal with skimmed milk, toasted seeded bread spread with peanut butter, a cooked breakfast (grilled lean bacon and low-fat sausages and poached eggs) served with baked beans in tomato sauce, kedgeree made with basmati rice.

Lunch can include a baked potato with baked beans in tomato sauce, seeded bread or rolls with lentil soup, sandwiches using seeded bread, baked beans on toast, bean and pasta salads, pita breads filled with salad.

The main meal can include roasted meats or baked fish served with large amounts of vegetables especially beans and new potatoes cooked in their skins, casseroles that include beans and chickpeas, pasta dishes served with extra vegetables and tomato sauces.

Low G.I. for the family

This is such a simple way of eating that the family will probably not notice that the foods have a low G.I. It is ideal for all family members as the meals are sustaining and satisfying and mean that everyone can get on with enjoying life rather than seeking out the next snack.

For children it is an especially good way of eating as it fills them up and thus stops them continually wanting sugary and salty snacks. Also the moderated and sustained blood sugar level may help concentration levels—and behavior.

Unfortunately many children are overweight these days and there are preliminary suggestions that a low-G.I. diet helps to prevent this.

For many elderly people the low-G.I. meals are evocative of traditional dishes containing more grains and legumes.

Shopping

When shopping for low-G.I. foods, look for fresh and dried fruits, vegetables, and legumes. Many people worry about soaking and cooking dried beans. If you are concerned, invest in lots of cans of these beans both for quickness and convenience. But do buy a pack of dried lentils, as they are so easy to cook and have a very low G.I. They do not require soaking, take only 15 minutes to cook, and make a wonderful addition to curries and casseroles.

● Any dried beans or split peas, and cereals like barley have a very low G.I. and the dried ones, when home-cooked, result in a final dish with a lower G.I. than if canned varieties are used.

● Look for seeded bread, or make your own in a bread maker, which is so easy to do. You can buy packs of seeds such as linseeds, sesame, pumpkin, and sunflower seeds which you can add to breads, rolls, stir-fries, and salads. You can even grow your own sunflowers and then use the seeds—if you do this, do not use any pesticide sprays.

● Invest in a large pack of oats to make oatmeal and add to muffins and crumbles and to thicken soups, casseroles, and tagines.

● Buy skim milk and low-fat yogurt for cooking, even if you are not keen on skim milk in teas and coffees. Make rice puddings and custards with them to provide a low-calorie and low-G.I. comfort food.

● Choose rapeseed oil (canola or lear oil) or olive oil in cooking and use a minimum of it. An oil-water spray may be useful to cut down on the amount of fat in cooking.

● Choose good-quality lean meat and a range of different types of fish and poultry.

● Invest in a wide range of herbs; the fresh ones are delicious and can be a basis for growing a garden at home. Also try a range of spices to flavor dishes.

Cooking

● The more highly processed the food, then the higher the G.I. Consider apples: a whole apple will have a lower G.I. than stewed apple or apple juice. The more breaking down that the body has to do to release the glucose from a food, then the lower the G.I. Try to keep foods as whole as possible, i.e., do not peel fruit and vegetables and try not to mash or puree them. If you are making soup, blend only half of it and enjoy the chunky textures.

● Try to use a minimum of spread on bread, and you may find that eating grain breads and rolls with their tasty, nutty flavor means that you do not need a spread at all.

● To reduce the calorie content of meals ensure that fat is trimmed from all meats and the skin is stripped from poultry before eating.

● Where a fat or oil is needed in cooking, use an oil spray or even a pastry brush to spread oil over the bottom of a pan or over potatoes or vegetables for roasting.

● Stir-fries can actually be cooked in a little water rather than oil to start them off.

● Dry-fry pans, which have a special lid or a shiny surface on the inside of the lid, can be used to brown meat or chunks of vegetables. Using such a reflective surface on a lid can even be used to fry eggs successfully. Just use a spray of oil or a brush full of oil in the pan to start the process.

● To keep the fat level of dishes down, make sure you bake, broil, steam, microwave, stew, or braise rather than deep-fat fry. Remember that batters and bread crumbs really absorb a lot of fat so avoid these coatings on fish and chicken, or oven bake them if they do tempt you.

● Limit the amount of salt in cooking by using a range of herbs and spices.

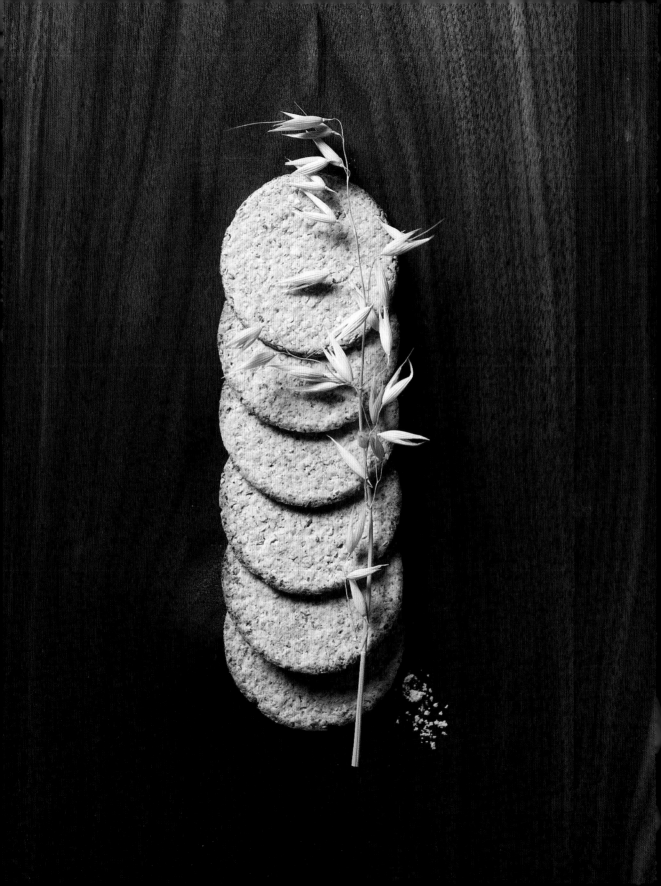

Packed lunches

Many of us have to take packed lunches, so eating a lunch with a lower G.I. will help to keep us from feeling hungry all afternoon. The resulting more moderate and sustained level of blood glucose will also make us feel more alert.

Choose a bean or pasta salad, use grain breads and rolls for sandwiches, have lentil and bean soups and follow these with fresh fruits, oat muffins, low-fat yogurts, seed cakes, peanuts, or slices of fruit breads.

Snacks

A quick bite to eat can be really useful in curbing hunger pangs, particularly for children, teenagers, those with digestive problems, and those involved in sport.

There are masses of high-fat and high-sugar snacks available and there is nothing wrong with these as an occasional treat.

However, to keep the G.I. levels down and thus promote a feeling of fullness, snacks such as unpeeled fresh fruit, peanuts, oatcakes, oat cookies, seeded bread and buns are much better.

You will find recipes for muffins and fruit breads as well as seeded rolls in this book, which are all excellent as snacks.

Convenience foods

When days are a rush it is useful to choose a chilled or frozen ready-made meal—indeed it can be a way of experimenting with new flavors which may tempt you to cook them yourself at a later date.

But, this "snip and ping" way of eating, where we snip open the package and put it in the microwave to await the ping that tells us it is ready, can be unbalanced as many of the foods can be high in fat and salt but with little fruit and vegetable content.

They are also often not very satisfying and the serving sizes can be small, so the nutritional information on the package is deceptive as you may end up eating the meal designed for two on your own. Compare these with the size you would serve at home if preparing fresh cooked dishes. The next time you make your own lasagne, make a larger quantity so you can freeze the extra and create your own healthy microwave meals.

However, served with extras such as some vegetables, new potatoes cooked in their skins, seeded breads or rolls or pasta, convenience foods can become a satisfying and balanced meal and one with a low G.I.

Fresh vegetables can be bought ready-prepared and take little time to cook, but a standby of bags of frozen vegetables is also valuable. They can be cooked in a microwave or quickly in a pan.

Eating out

It does not matter where you eat out—whether a fast-food or a deluxe restaurant—the same principles apply as at home for reducing the G.I. level of meals.

● Choose grainy breads and rolls in preference to white or whole-wheat; if the restaurant does not serve those, perhaps asking will stimulate them to do so.

● Choose chunky vegetable or lentil soups rather than smooth creamy ones.

● For main courses, select broiled or grilled meat, fish, or poultry, or a low-fat vegetarian dish. Choose those entrées to be served with beans or peas for greater satisfaction.

● Pasta dishes with a tomato-based sauce, and beans can be an excellent way of reducing the G.I. level of main courses.

● Indian meals with lentils, chickpeas, and beans are all naturally low in G.I. but may be high in fat so ask for them to be cooked without fat.

Select items on the menu with a lower calorie content, e.g., those without a pastry crust, creamy sauces, and which have not been fried, and accompany these with lots of vegetables. Ask for the vegetables to be served without any butter.

For dessert, choose a fruit-based pudding, sherbert, or ice cream. If you choose a higher calorie dessert that comes with cream or ice cream, opt for the ice cream.

As the final tip for eating out: try to curb the amount of alcohol and thus keep the calorie level down by drinking lots of water.

Fast foods and take-out meals

When you are rushing around or traveling, it is often tempting to grab a burger or pizza for a quick snack. That quick snack, though, can often leave you looking for another meal so try to plan in advance what you will eat, or choose carefully from the fast-food or take-out menu.

Choose a seeded bun with your burger and avoid the mayo to save calories. And eat just a half-portion of fries with your burger.

Choose pizzas topped with vegetables rather than pepperoni, extra cheese, or ham.

Pasta is ideal provided a tomato rather than a creamy sauce accompanies it.

Indian food with its range of legumes is ideal; just ask for the dish to be made with less fat and avoid the obviously fried items such as onion pakoras, samosas, and fried rice. Opt for plain boiled rice, ask for the poppadoms to be cooked in a microwave rather than deep-fried, have a side dish of dal to fill up on, and avoid the kormas because of the coconut cream they contain.

At the Chinese take-out restaurant, avoid fried rice and items such as battered sweet and sour shrimp and opt for dishes with noodles, plain rice, and plenty of vegetables.

Most restaurants now offer a range of salads and those containing beans and corn are particularly useful thanks to their low G.I.

Choose whole fruit or chunky fruits as dessert. Opt for low-fat ice cream and at least avoid the whipped cream with ordinary sundaes.

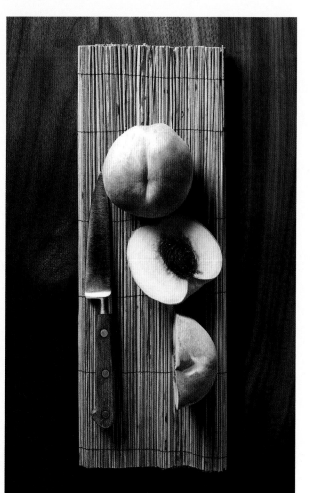

menu planning

These wonderful recipes that Antony has created provide a delicious basis for meals. They are a brilliant blend of ingredients with a low G.I. as well as being low in calories. The recipes are also low in fat, salt, and sugar, and include large portions of vegetables and fruit, thus reflecting the guidelines for healthy eating.

All the recipes are straightforward and easy to prepare and can be included in family eating. The use of different ingredients is inspirational and encourages the cook to try other recipes as well as developing their own variations.

Portion sizes

One of the marvelous things about the recipes is that they offer really substantial portions. Unlike most other diets, you will find each meal really satisfying and won't crave extra food and snacks.

About the nutritional calculations

The recipes have been calculated to show the calories per portion. They also show the amount of fat and saturated fat per portion in grams. The sodium content of recipes per portion is also shown.

All of the recipes have been calculated based on the smallest number of portions, for example, if a recipe makes 4–6 portions, the nutritional breakdown has been calculated for 4 portions.

Where salt is included in the recipe, we have allowed for ¼ teaspoon (2g) per 4 portions.

The majority of the recipes have been created to provide under 300 calories per portion to help you lose weight at a sensible rate. Once you have achieved your target weight, there are a number of recipes that are between 300 and 500 calories per portion (indicated by a green semi-circle at the top of the recipe).

Serving suggestions

These are given with most of the recipes and are an integral part of the diet. Not only do they complement the dish, they will also reduce the G.I. of the meal, so do please take note of them. Of course, you can alter them to suit your tastes, but try to add vegetables, potatoes in their skins, brown rice, noodles, pasta, or grainy bread to each meal.

Menu planners

These menu planners have been put together based on the recipes from the book. They give an idea of how to eat a satisfying and healthy diet which is also low in calories and can thus help weight loss or weight maintenance. The menus allow for extra fruit and vegetables as well as a scraping of butter or low-fat spreads on bread. However, with seeded bread, people often find they do not need the butter as the bread is so tasty. Also there is a daily allowance made for 2¼ cups of skim or 2% milk in teas or coffees.

Plenty of fluid is also recommended as is water and diluted juices. Even the odd glass of wine can be included.

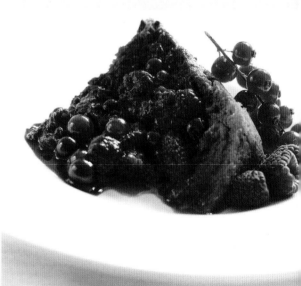

Menu 1

Breakfast
Egg White Omelet
1 slice of South African Seed Bread

Mid-Morning
Apple

Lunch
2 slices of South African Seed Bread with
  Lentil Spread
Herbed Leaf Salad

Red Fruits

Mid-Afternoon
Pear

Dinner
Pan-Fried Mullet with Olives and
  Tomatoes
New Potatoes
Green Beans

Rice Pudding

Snack
Scotch Pancakes and Honey

Plenty of fluids throughout the day

Menu 2

Breakfast
Oatmeal with Berries

Mid-Morning
Banana

Lunch
Leek and Pea Soup

Simple Roast Chicken
Baked Sweet Potatoes and Roasted
  Vegetables
Broccoli

Summer Pudding (see page 140)
Low-Fat Fromage Frais or Yogurt

Mid-Afternoon
Carrot and Pineapple Cake

Dinner
Argula, Belgian Endive and Parmesan
  Salad
Barley and Goat Cheese Soufflé Bake

Whole Poached Apricots

Snack
Soda Bread Roll
Carrot Cocktail

Plenty of fluids throughout the day

Menu 3

Breakfast
Caribbean Smoothie

Mid-Morning
Blueberry Muffin

Lunch
Smoked Salmon (Lox) and Cottage
  Cheese Sandwich
2 plums

Mid-Afternoon
Plain Low-Fat Yogurt with Cherries

Dinner
Thai Fish Cakes with Cucumber Relish
Large Green Salad with Beans
Fresh Fruit Salad

Snack
1 slice of Orange and Almond Cake

Plenty of fluids throughout the day

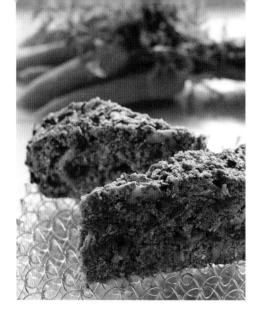

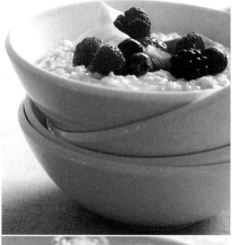

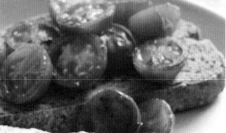

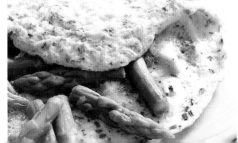

breakfasts and baking

blueberry muffins

Blueberries are wonderfully versatile fruits. They are great eaten fresh or cooked in pies or muffins and if you have a surplus in season, freeze them quickly and they won't lose their valuable nutrients. Fresh blueberries are one of the best sources of vitamin C.

MAKES 9 SMALL MUFFINS

Scant 2 cups whole-grain flour
2 teaspoons baking powder
2 tablespoons raw cane sugar
2/3 cup skim milk
1 medium egg
2 tablespoons vegetable oil
1 1/3 cup blueberries—fresh or frozen

1 Preheat the oven to 350°F.

2 Line nine cups of a muffin tray with paper muffin cups.

3 Mix the flour, baking powder, and sugar together in a large mixing bowl.

4 In a separate bowl, whisk the milk, egg, and oil together. Make a well in the center of the flour and quickly fold in the liquid, then add the blueberries.

5 Divide the mixture among the muffin cups and bake for 25–30 minutes until risen and golden. You can test whether the muffins are cooked by lightly pressing one; if the top springs back, they are ready.

Per muffin: 141 cal., 4g fat, 0.5g sat. fat, 0.15g sodium, 23g carbohydrate

oatmeal with berries

There is no better way to start the day than with a hot bowl of oatmeal. This is a really low-G.I. breakfast, especially compared to breakfast cereals, and will keep you satisfied until lunch, so no need for croissants at coffee time.

SERVES 6

2 cups medium oatmeal or rolled oats
Pinch of salt
1/2 teaspoon ground cinnamon
Low-fat plain yogurt, for serving
12 ounces berries of your choice, fresh or frozen (such as strawberries, blackberries, raspberries, blueberries)—about 2–3 cups

1 Put 5 cups water on to boil in a large saucepan. When it comes to a boil, slowly pour in the oats, stirring continuously. Reduce the heat to a level where the surface of the oatmeal faintly "burps." Stir in the salt and cinnamon.

2 Let cook until the oatmeal has reached the desired consistency—this will take about 15 minutes for a sloppy texture or 20 minutes for a firmer one.

3 Spoon the oatmeal into six bowls, place a good spoonful of yogurt on top, then add a ladleful of berries.

Per portion: 162 cal., 3g fat, 0.2g sat. fat, 0.07g sodium, 29g carbohydrate

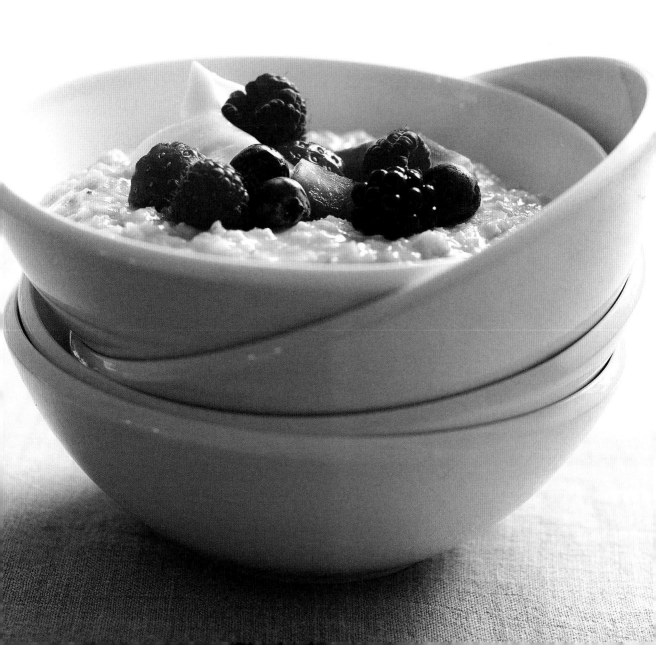

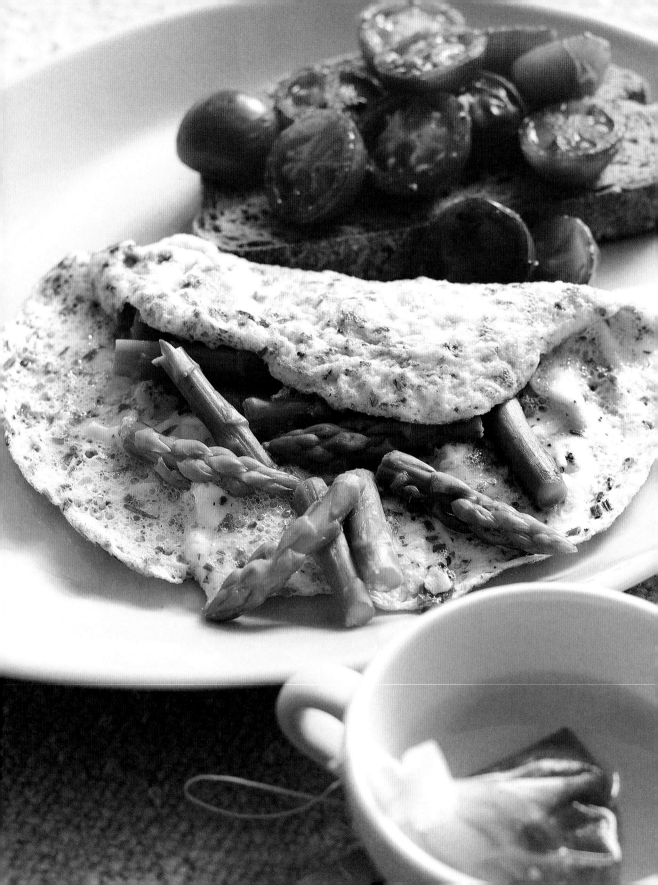

egg white omelet with asparagus and herbs

By using only the egg whites in this omelet, you remove almost all the fat content of the egg, as that is concentrated in the yolk. The easiest way to separate an egg is to crack it open and pour the white into a bowl, while catching the yolk in the shell.

SERVES 1

Small pat of unsalted butter
3 egg whites (keep yolks for another use)
1 tablespoon finely chopped herbs such as chives, tarragon, or chervil
Salt and ground black pepper
6 thin asparagus spears, cooked and cut into 1-inch sections and kept warm
Whole-grain bread, toasted
Cherry tomatoes

1 Heat the butter in a small nonstick omelet pan over medium heat.

2 Whisk the egg whites with a fork and add the herbs, a pinch of salt, and ground black pepper. Pour the egg white into the omelet pan and with a fork, quickly pull the edges to the center, so the omelet cooks evenly.

3 When cooked but still creamy, place the warm asparagus in the center and leave on the heat for a second longer. Then fold the omelet in half, giving the pan a light tap to loosen the omelet. Slide out onto a warm plate. Serve with whole-grain toast and some warmed cherry tomatoes.

Per portion: 154 cal., 10g fat, 5.9g sat. fat, 0.38g sodium, 3g carbohydrate

breakfast kitcheri

A kitcheri is a traditional Indian vegetarian dish that evolved into kedgeree, an Anglo-Indian favorite. This recipe is a fusion of both, combining the lentils in kitcheri with fish from kedgeree. The result is a low-G.I. dish that is perfect for brunch or supper.

SERVES 4

9 ounces kippered herring, smoked haddock or salmon fillet
1 1/4 cups skim milk
1 bay leaf
1 small onion, chopped
2 teaspoons unsalted butter
1 tablespoon curry paste
1 1/3 cups cooked brown basmati rice
One x 15-ounce can lentils (or 1 3/4 cups cooked lentils), drained and rinsed
2 hard-boiled eggs, chopped
2 tablespoons chopped parsley
Ground black pepper

1 Cook your chosen combination of fish in the milk with the bay leaf over medium heat for 5–7 minutes, then set aside to let cool slightly.

2 Meanwhile, cook the onion slowly in the butter until soft but not browned, then add the curry paste and stir to combine.

3 Strain the milk and set aside. Remove the fish from the pan and flake it, discarding the skin and bones and the bay leaf.

4 Add the rice and lentils to the onion and heat through, then add the flaked fish, hard-boiled eggs, and parsley, and stir. Add enough of the reserved milk (about 2/3 cup) to make the mixture luscious and moist, then season to taste with black pepper and serve immediately.

Per portion: 418 cal., 20g fat, 4.9g sat. fat, 0.66g sodium, 36g carbohydrate

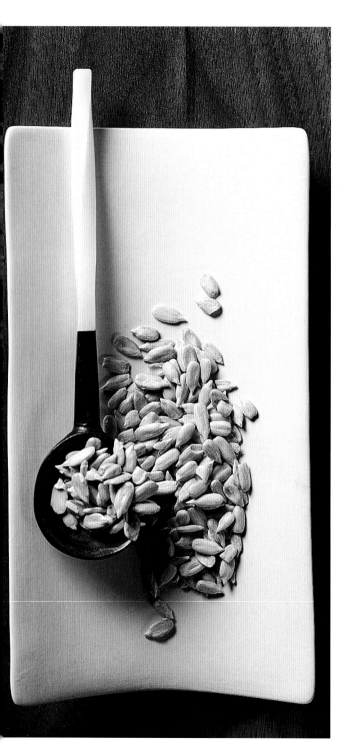

muesli mix

Muesli is one of the healthiest ways to start the day. Store-bought versions may contain added sugar, so it is well worth taking the time to make your own. You can vary the choice of nuts, seeds, and fruit—try adding linseeds, which are a good source of omega-3 fatty acids.

SERVES 10

2^1/4 cups rolled oats
4 cups bran flakes
3 tablespoons wheat germ
^{1}/4 cup sunflower seeds
^{1}/4 cup raisins or golden raisins
^{1}/2 cup hazelnuts or Brazil nuts, roughly chopped
1 cup dried fruits such as pears, figs, apricots, chopped

Combine all the ingredients and store in an airtight container.

Per portion: 236 cal., 7g fat, 0.4g sat. fat, 0.10g sodium, 38g carbohydrate

apple and hazelnut muesli

This will keep in the fridge for 2–3 days. Add extra fruit juice or yogurt as required to give a spoonable consistency. You can add extra berries or chopped fruit.

SERVES 3–4

1 cup rolled oats
1 cup very low-fat plain yogurt
^{2}/3 cup apple juice
2 pink-skinned apples, such as gala, cored and
   coarsely grated
^{1}/4 cup chopped toasted hazelnuts

Combine all the ingredients together until well mixed.

Per portion: 298 cal., 9g fat, 0.8g sat. fat, 0.09g sodium, 46g carboyhdrate

tropical fruit shake

This is a really thick shake and a great way to get kids to increase their fruit intake. You can use either fresh or frozen tropical fruit, varying the choice depending upon season or tastes.

SERVES 2

4 ounces tropical fruit, chopped (about 3/4 cup)
1 medium-ripe banana
1 tablespoon honey
2/3 cup skim milk
2/3 cup orange juice
1/4 cup low-fat plain yogurt

Blend all the ingredients in a blender. If using fresh fruit or if the fruit has defrosted, you may want to add 3–4 ice cubes.

Pour into tall glasses for serving.

Per portion: 200 cal., 2g fat, 0.6g sat. fat, 0.13g sodium, 41g carbohydrate

caribbean smoothie

Here's a rich, luxurious breakfast drink. The addition of the bran increases the fiber content.

SERVES 4–6

3 bananas, peeled and chopped
2 cups pineapple juice
1 1/4 cups skim milk
2 tablespoons coconut cream
2 tablespoons bran

Blend all the ingredients in a blender until smooth enough to drink. Add extra juice or milk as necessary to create the perfect consistency. Pour into tall glasses for serving.

Per portion: 193 cal., 5g fat, 3.9g sat. fat, 0.05g sodium, 35g carbohydrate

mountain bread

For a plain version, simply omit the garlic and spices.

SERVES 16 – MAKES 32 SLICES

1 pound whole-grain flour (about 3^1/$_3$ cups)
10^1/$_2$ ounces semolina (about 2^1/$_4$ cups)
2 teaspoons salt
^{3}/$_4$ teaspoon cayenne pepper
1^1/$_4$ tablespoons garlic, crushed—about 1 medium head
^{1}/$_2$ teaspoon chili powder
^{1}/$_2$ teaspoon ground black pepper
^{1}/$_2$ teaspoon paprika
Vegetable oil, for greasing
2 egg yolks, beaten
^{1}/$_2$ cup sunflower seeds
3 tablespoons poppy seeds

1 Preheat the oven to 425°F.

2 Mix together all the dry ingredients and place in a food-processor with a dough hook fitted. With the machine running on a slow speed, gradually add 2 cups warm water (from a tea kettle) until a dough forms. Let the machine run for 5–8 minutes to knead well.

3 Break the dough into eight pieces and either put it through a pasta machine or roll out to ^{1}/$_8$-inch-thick strips. Cut each piece into four. Place the dough pieces on lightly oiled nonstick baking sheets and brush lightly with egg yolk, then sprinkle liberally with the seeds. Bake for about 15 minutes or until golden, remove, and let cool for 5 minutes then transfer to a wire rack. Store in an airtight container.

Per 2 slices: 190 cal., 4g fat, 0.5g sat. fat, 0.25g sodium, 38g carbohydrate

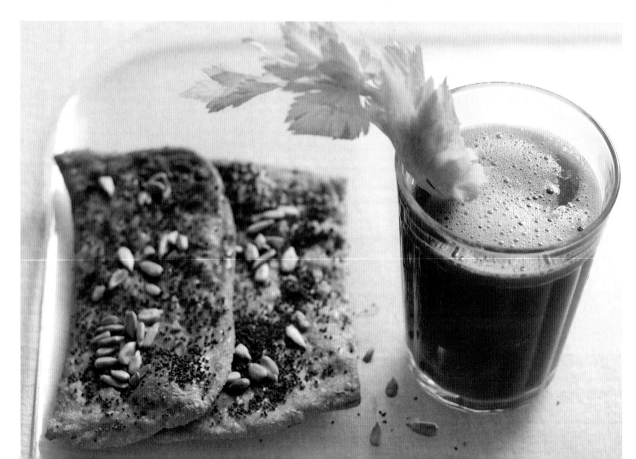

carrot cocktail

Give your immune system a boost with this revitalizing drink (photographed bottom left). Carrots provide lots of beta carotene, which acts as an antioxidant and is a substance the body can change into vitamin A. The ginger will help digestion and fight off colds.

SERVES 1–2

1¼ cups organic carrot juice
½-inch piece of fresh ginger root, peeled
1 stalk of celery, sliced lengthwise

1 Put all the ingredients into a blender and whizz until smooth. Pour it over some crushed ice and serve with a stalk of celery in each glass.

2 Serve with mountain bread (see opposite page) or a whole-grain bread roll.

Per portion: 80 cal., 0.4g fat, 0g sat. fat, 0.18g sodium, 19g carbohydrate

whole-grain soda bread or rolls

If you use milk instead of yogurt or buttermilk in this recipe you will only need to use about 1½ cups.

MAKES 1 LOAF (8 WEDGES) OR 16 ROLLS

18 ounces whole-grain brown flour (about 3¾ cups)
1 teaspoon salt
1½ teaspoons baking soda
1 teaspoon sugar
About 1¾ cups skim milk, low-fat plain yogurt
   or buttermilk

1 Preheat the oven to 450°F.

2 Stir the dry ingredients together in a mixing bowl. Make a well in the center and pour in 1½ cups milk or 1¾ cups yogurt or buttermilk.

3 Using one hand in a circular motion, mix in the flour to form a dough which is softish without being too wet or sticky—add more milk or flour if necessary. Turn the dough out onto a floured board. Knead just enough to tidy the dough into a neat ball.

4 For bread, pat the dough into a circle 1½ inches deep and cut a deep cross on the surface. Bake for 15 minutes on a floured baking tray, then reduce the heat to 400°F for another 25–30 minutes. For rolls, cut the dough into 16 pieces. Bake for about 20 minutes at the higher temperature.

5 To test whether it is cooked, tap the bottom of the bread and if it sounds hollow, it is ready.

Per wedge or 2 rolls: 108 cal., 1g fat, 0.1g sat. fat, 0.24g sodium, 22g carbohydrate

scotch pancakes

These thick pancakes are also known as drop scones. Serve with fresh fruit and a light drizzle of honey.

SERVES 4 – MAKES 12

^{1}/$_3$ cup whole-grain flour
^{1}/$_3$ cup all-purpose flour
^{1}/$_2$ teaspoon cream of tartar
^{1}/$_2$ teaspoon baking soda
1 teaspoon sugar
1 medium egg, preferably free-range
^{1}/$_4$–^{1}/$_2$ cup 2% or low-fat milk

1 Put the whole-grain flour in a bowl then sift in the rest of the dry ingredients. Make a well in the center with a wooden spoon and add the egg. Break the yolk and pour in the milk, mixing quickly to a thick batter. Do not beat, as this develops the gluten in the flour and prevents the pancakes from rising.

2 Fry spoonfuls of the mixture in a lightly greased, hot skillet or heavy frying pan for 1–2 minutes on each side until risen and golden and springy to the touch. Serve warm.

Per portion: 120 cal., 2g fat, 0.8g sat. fat, 0.17g sodium, 20g carbohydrate

passion fruit curd

Extremely simple to make, this delicious fruit preserve is great with whole-grain toast or oat cakes. It also makes a terrific gift, so if you see passion fruit going cheap why not buy in bulk and make a big batch?

SERVES 10 – MAKES 300ML (1¼ CUPS)

^{1}/$_2$ cup sugar
^{1}/$_4$ cup (^{1}/$_2$ stick) unsalted butter
2 eggs, beaten
6 passion fruit, pulp and seeds

1 Stir the sugar with the unsalted butter in a nonstick saucepan over medium heat until the sugar has dissolved.

2 Add the eggs and the passion fruit pulp and seeds, stirring continuously over the gentlest of heat for about 10 minutes until thickened. Do not let it boil. If preferred, use a double boiler.

3 Pour into a sterilized jar and refrigerate for up to 2 months.

Per portion: 108 cal., 6g fat, 3.5g sat. fat, 0.02g sodium, 12g carbohydrate

orange and almond cake

This moist cake has a texture reminiscent of baked cheesecake. Keep in the fridge in an airtight container and eat within 3–4 days.

SERVES 12–16

2 large thin-skinned oranges
1 cup caster sugar
7 ounces ground almonds (about 2¼ cups)
½ teaspoon baking powder
6 eggs
Juice of ½ lemon

1 Put the oranges in a pan and cover with cold water. Bring to a boil, reduce the heat, cover, and simmer for 2 hours. Top up with water if necessary so that they are always covered. Remove from the water and let cool.

2 Preheat the oven to 350°F. Grease and line a 9-inch cake pan.

3 Cut the oranges into chunks and remove any seeds. Put the oranges in a food processor with all the remaining ingredients and blend until well mixed. Transfer the batter to the prepared pan and bake for 45–60 minutes until risen and firm to the touch. Cool, then transfer to a wire rack.

Per slice: 223 cal., 13g fat, 1.7g sat. fat, 0.06g sodium, 22g carbohydrate

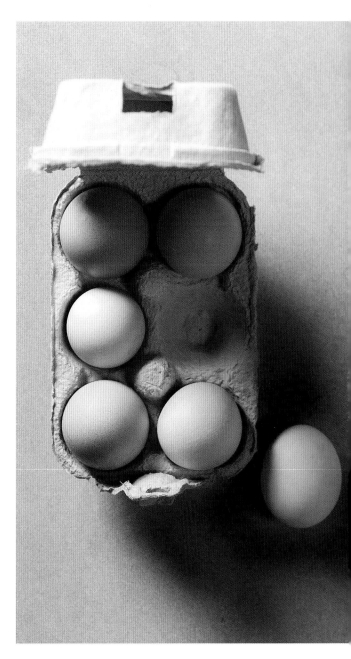

south african seed bread

This bread has an extremely low G.I. as the tough outer coating of the seeds makes them harder to break down. The seeds are also excellent sources of omega-3 fatty acids and phytoestrogens. Quick to mix and only one rising required, this heavily seeded bread always has a fairly flat top.

MAKES 2 LOAVES – 18 SLICES EACH

1 pound, 6 ounces whole-grain flour (about 4³/4–5 cups)
1/2 cup bran
1/4-oz. envelope, fast-action (rapid-rise) yeast
1/2 cup sunflower seeds
1/2 cup sesame seeds
1/2 cup pumpkin seeds
1/2 cup linseeds
2 tablespoons dark brown sugar
1 teaspoon salt
2 tablespoons vegetable oil

1 Grease 2-pound loaf pans (8¹/2-inches long). Mix the flour, bran, yeast, seeds, sugar, and salt in a large bowl. Add the oil and 2¹/2 cups hand-hot water and mix to a soft dough.

2 Divide the mixture between the pans, cover with a oiled plastic wrap, and let rise in a warm place until the mixture reaches the top of the pans (this will take 30–60 minutes).

3 Meanwhile, preheat the oven to 400°F and bake the loaves in the center of the oven for about 40 minutes until risen and firm to the touch. Once cooked the loaves will sound hollow when tapped on the bottom. Cool on wire racks.

Per slice: 100 cal., 4g fat, 0.5g sat. fat, 0.06g sodium, 13g carbohydrate

carrot and pineapple cake

This is a moist, luscious cake filled with carrots, nuts, and spices—a real treat. It also freezes well.

SERVES 16

1 pound whole-wheat flour (about 3¹/3 cups)
2 tablespoons baking powder
1¹/2 teaspoons salt
1/2 tablespoon ground cinnamon
1/2 teaspoon ground nutmeg
1/2 teaspoon ground allspice
1/2 cup dark brown sugar
1/2 cup light olive oil
2 eggs, lightly beaten
12 ounces carrot, grated (about 2¹/2 cups)
1/2 cup walnut pieces
1/2 cup raisins
1/2 cup dry, unsweetened coconut
9 ounces crushed pineapple in natural juice (about 1 cup)
Confectioners' sugar, for dusting (optional)

1 Preheat the oven to 350°F. Grease and line the bottom of a 9-inch springform pan with parchment paper. (If you have no parchment paper, then grease and flour the pan's bottom.)

2 Mix all the dry ingredients together in a large bowl. Add the remaining ingredients except the confectioners' sugar and mix well until evenly combined.

3 Transfer the batter to the prepared pan and level the surface. Bake in the center of the oven for about 1 hour until risen and golden and a fine metal skewer comes out clean when inserted in the cake.

4 Cool in the pan for 15 minutes, then transfer to a wire rack until completely cold. Dust with confectioners' sugar before serving.

Per slice: 259 cal., 13g fat, 2.5g sat. fat, 0.08g sodium, 34g carbohydrate

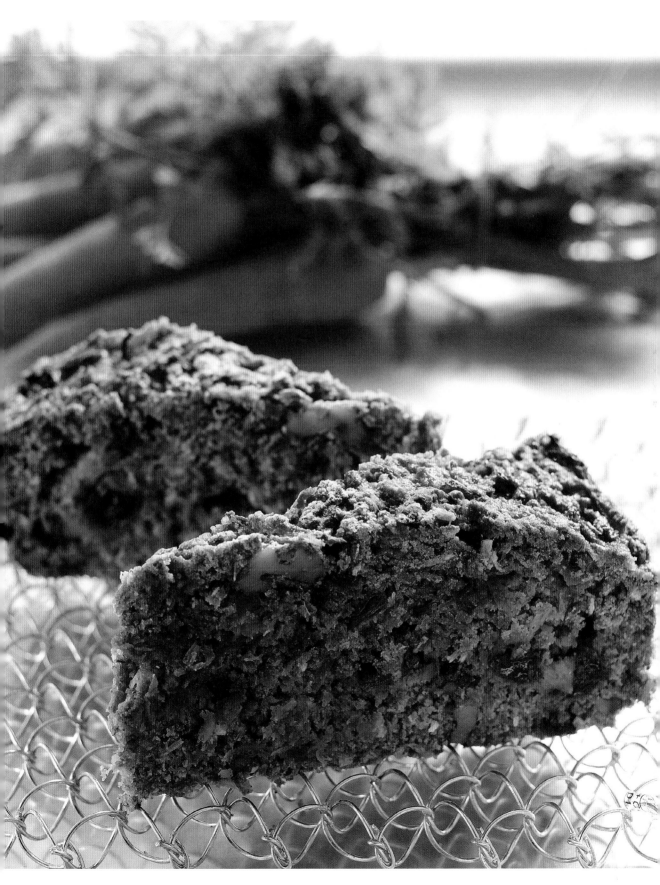

fruited tea bread

Moist loaves packed full of dried fruit—a slice makes a
perfect snack. You need to soak the raisins and golden
raisins in hot tea overnight.

MAKES 2 LOAVES – 16 SLICES PER LOAF

7 ounces golden raisins (about 1¹/3 cups)

7 ounces raisins (about 1¹/3 cups)

2 cups hot tea

12 ounces whole-wheat flour (about 2¹/2 cups)

2 teaspoons apple pie spice

2 teaspoons baking powder

¹/4 cup light brown sugar

6 ounces dates (about 1 cup), chopped

²/3 cup dried apricots, chopped

2 tablespoons butter, melted

2 eggs, beaten

1 Soak the raisins and golden raisins in the tea overnight.

2 Preheat the oven to 325°F.

3 Grease 2 x 1-pound (6-inch-long) loaf pans and line the
bottoms with parchment paper. (If you have no parchment
paper, then grease and flour the bottom.)

4 Place all the dry ingredients in a large bowl and mix well.
Add the soaked fruit with any extra liquid, and the remaining
ingredients and mix well. Divide between the pans and level
the surface.

5 Bake for 50–60 minutes until risen and firm to the touch.
Cool in the pans then transfer to a wire rack until cold.

**Per slice: 98 cal., 1g fat, 0.6g sat. fat, 0.05g sodium,
21g carbohydrate**

finnish barley bread

This is an unusual bread—with a crisp outer crust and a
dense moist center—perfect for anyone trying to cut
out wheat. Great with soup or cheese.

MAKES 1 FLAT LOAF – 16 SLICES

14 ounces (about 2 cups) barley

2¹/4 cups buttermilk

Vegetable oil, for greasing

9 ounces (about 1³/4 cups) barley flour, plus a little extra

1 teaspoon baking powder

1 teaspoon salt

1 Combine the barley and buttermilk in a medium-sized
bowl, cover, and let soak overnight.

2 Preheat the oven to 350°F.

3 Lightly oil and flour an 8- to 9-inch cast-iron frying pan.

4 Add 1 cup water to the buttermilk and barley mixture,
then transfer to the blender and blend until the barley is well
pulverized (it will not become a smooth puree).

5 Return this batter to the bowl, add the barley flour, baking
powder, and salt, and mix well. Spoon the batter into the
frying pan. Bake in the center of the oven for about 1 hour.
Let cool on a wire rack before serving.

**Per slice: 158 cal., 1g fat, 0.2g sat. fat, 0.17g sodium,
36g carbohydrate**

dried fruit compote

Another great way to begin your day with a good helping of fruit and nuts. This low-G.I. breakfast will prevent you feeling hungry during the morning.

SERVES 4

^{2}/$_3$ cups small dried apricots
^{1}/$_3$ cup dried cherries
^{1}/$_3$ cup dried blueberries
5 dried figs, cut in half
^{1}/$_3$ cup dried pears, cut in half
^{1}/$_3$ cup dried mango, cut into bite-sized pieces
^{1}/$_2$ cinnamon stick
2 cloves
^{1}/$_2$ vanilla bean, split
Finely grated zest of ^{1}/$_2$ lemon
Pinch saffron
1^1/$_2$ tablespoons slivered almonds, toasted
1^1/$_2$ tablespoons pine nuts
Few drops orange or rose water (optional)

1 Place all the ingredients down to and including the saffron in a non-reactive saucepan and just cover with cold water. Bring to a boil, reduce the heat, and simmer for 15 minutes.

2 Let cool then add the remaining ingredients. Serve with cereal, wheat germ, or low-fat plain yogurt.

Per portion: 189 cal., 5g fat, 0.4g sat. fat, 0.03g sodium, 34g carbohydrate

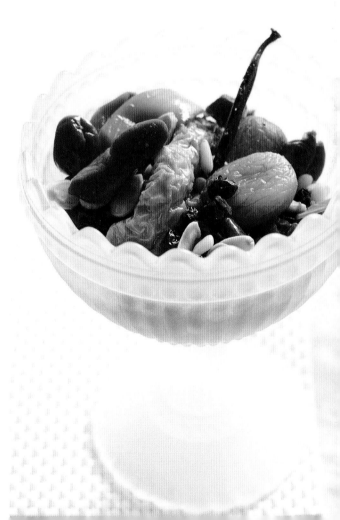

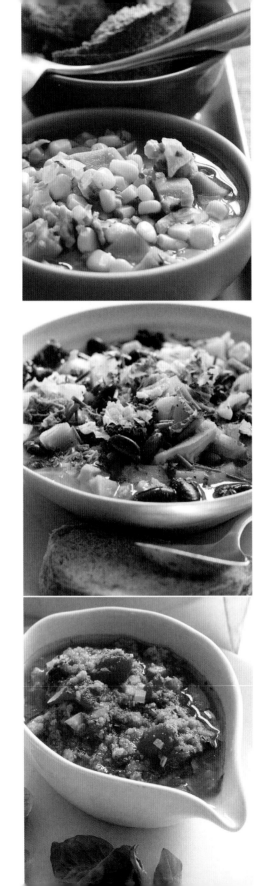

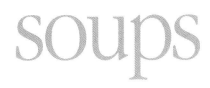

garlic soup with white beans

This is literally a heart-warming soup because while garlic has long been used as a protection against evil creatures, it has more recently been found to have medicinal qualities. Not only is it antibacterial, it will also boost your immune system and help prevent blood from clotting. Garlic is full of minerals and vitamins, too. Serve with whole-grain bread.

SERVES 6

2 large heads garlic, cloves separated and finely sliced
2 onions, finely chopped
1 teaspoon soft thyme leaves
2 tablespoons unsalted butter
1/4 cup cornstarch
6 cups chicken or vegetable broth
One x 15-ounce can of cannellini or navy beans (canned in water)
1 tablespoon red wine vinegar
Ground black pepper
Chopped fresh parsley or chives, for serving

1 In a large heavy pot, cook the garlic, onions, and thyme in the butter over medium heat until softened, adding a little broth if necessary to prevent sticking—this should take about 7 minutes. Reduce the heat, stir in the cornstarch and cook until lightly browned.

2 Add the broth gradually, stirring to avoid lumps. Increase the heat, bring to a boil and simmer for 30 minutes.

3 In small batches, pour the soup into a blender and blend until smooth. Return to the heat.

4 Drain and rinse the beans and add to the soup with the vinegar. Warm through. Season with black pepper and serve immediately sprinkled with herbs.

Per portion: 121 cal., 4g fat, 2.2g sat. fat, 0.20g sodium, 17g carbohydrate

tuscan tomato and bread soup

A rich, rustic Italian soup, where the bread reduces the G.I. of the overall meal. This is actually a meal in itself, so serve as a main course rather than an appetizer.

SERVES 6

1 tablespoon olive oil
1 onion, finely chopped
2 garlic cloves, crushed
2 1/4 pounds ripe tomatoes, peeled, seeded, and chopped (about 3 1/2–4 1/2 cups)
One x 14 1/2-ounce can of chopped tomatoes
4 thick slices whole-grain bread, roughly broken
Bunch of fresh basil
Ground black pepper

1 Heat the oil in a large pot. Add the onion and garlic and fry gently until the onion is soft but not brown.

2 Add the fresh tomatoes and cook for 1 minute. Add the canned tomatoes, bread, and basil, reserving a few basil leaves.

3 Simmer for 15 minutes stirring occasionally, adding up to 2 1/2 cups water to give a "sloppy" consistency. Just before serving, season with pepper and fold in the reserved basil leaves.

Per portion: 146 cal., 4g fat, 0.6g sat. fat, 0.22g sodium, 25g carbohydrate

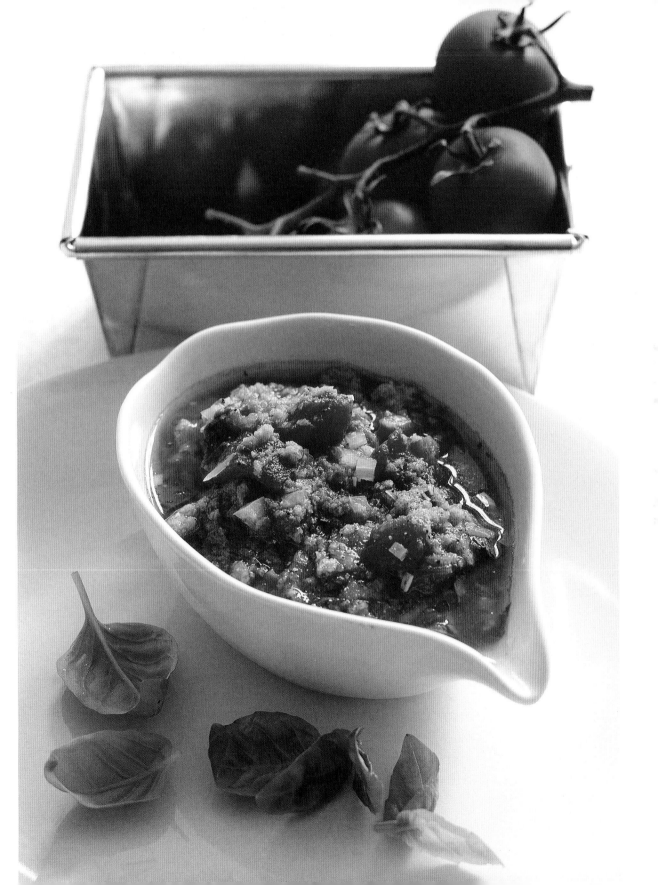

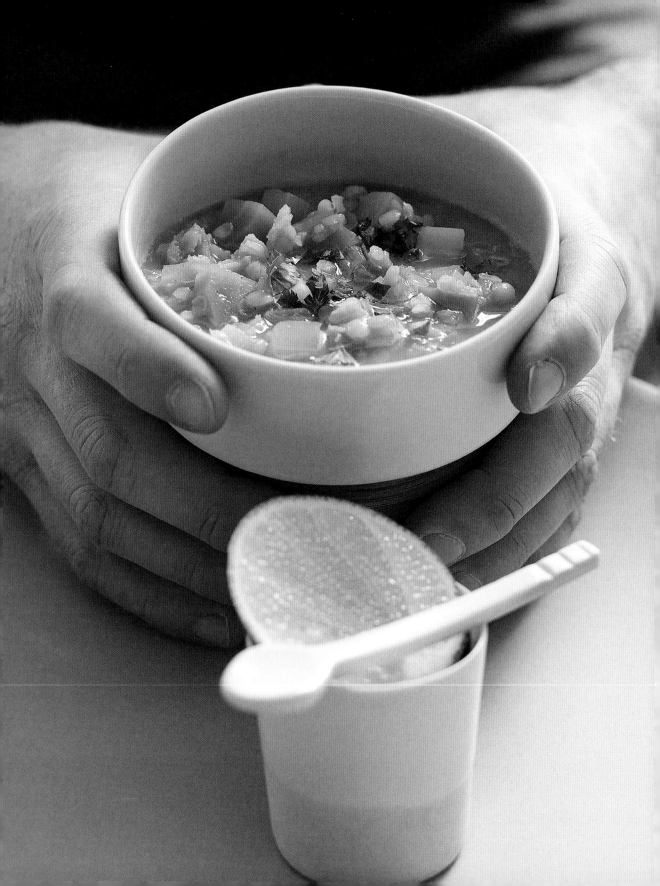

fragrant indian carrot and lentil soup

I have given a classic vegetarian soup a bit of a spicy twist, adding ginger, coriander, and curry powder. Blending only half the soup keeps the G.I. low and gives it texture.

SERVES 6–8

2 teaspoons unsalted butter
1 1/2 tablespoons grated fresh peeled ginger root
1/2 teaspoon each ground allspice, cumin, and chili powder
1/2 teaspoon curry powder
1/2 teaspoon ground coriander
2 onions, finely chopped
1 parsnip, chopped (if unavailable, add another 1 1/2 cups carrots)
1 stalk of celery, chopped
18 ounces carrots, sliced (about 4–5 cups)
1 cup red lentils, washed
1/4 cup brown basmati rice
8 cups vegetable broth
One x 14-ounce can of reduced-fat coconut milk
2 tablespoons fresh lime juice
3 tablespoons chopped fresh cilantro

1 Melt the butter in a heavy saucepan, add the ginger, allspice, cumin, chili powder, curry powder, and ground coriander. Cook over medium heat for 3 minutes.

2 Add the vegetables, stir to combine, and cook for another 8 minutes. Add the lentils and rice and stir in, before adding the broth. Bring to a boil and simmer for 30 minutes or until the vegetables are tender and the lentils have started to break down.

3 Blend half the soup in a blender or food processor until smooth. Return to the rest of the mixture, and add the coconut milk, lime juice, and cilantro. Heat through but do not let it boil again—this is important. Serve immediately.

Per portion: 215 cal., 3g fat, 1.6g sat. fat, 0.31g sodium, 39g carbohydrate

borlotti bean (cranberry bean) and cabbage soup

Borlotti (cranberry beans) are Italian beans traditionally used in stews and soups. They have a lovely smooth, slightly sweet taste that will enrich this thick winter soup.

SERVES 6

2 tablespoons extra-virgin olive oil
1 onion, finely chopped
3 garlic cloves, finely chopped
2 bay leaves
1 teaspoon fresh thyme leaves
1 chile, seeded and finely chopped
1/4 cup roughly chopped flat-leaf parsley
1 tablespoon chopped fresh marjoram
One x 14 1/2-ounce can of chopped tomatoes
Two x 15-ounce cans of cranberry beans (canned in water), drained and rinsed
3 cups vegetable broth
1 pound shredded greens (savoy cabbage, cavolo nero, spring greens)
Ground black pepper
Freshly grated Parmesan (optional)

1 Heat the olive oil in a large pot over medium heat, add the onion, garlic, bay leaves, thyme, and chile. Cook for about 10 minutes or until the onion has softened but is still colorless.

2 Add the herbs and tomatoes and cook for 3 minutes. Add the beans, broth, and 2 1/2 cups of water and cook for 30 minutes at a steady simmer.

3 Add the shredded greens and cook for 10 minutes. Thin as needed with extra water. Season to taste with black pepper. Pour into bowls and sprinkle with grated Parmesan, if you wish.

Per portion: 163 cal., 5g fat, 0.7g sat. fat, 0.45g sodium, 21g carbohydrate

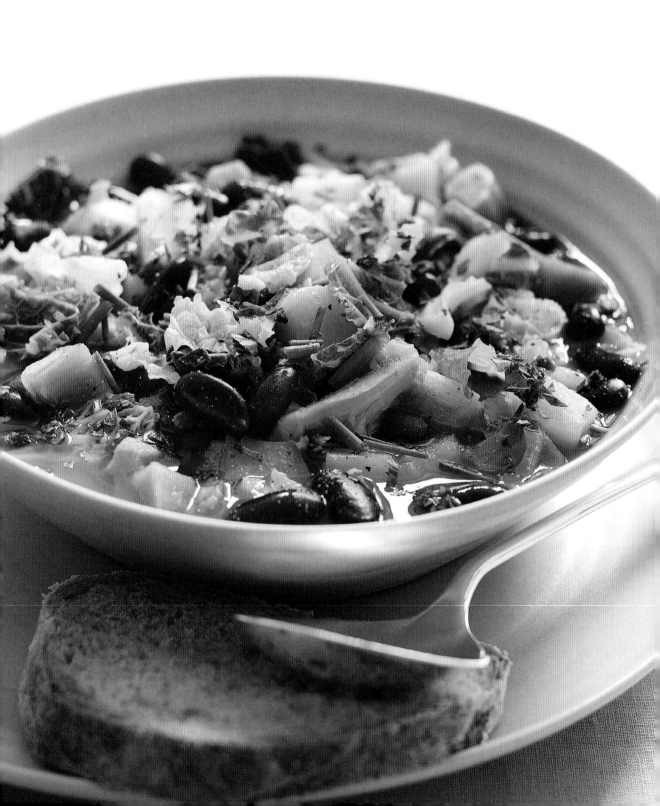

health in a bowl

The title says it all. I have thrown in every healthy ingredient I can think of and waved my magic spoon.

SERVES 8

1 pound thick-cut ham on the bone, chopped
2 1/2 quarts (10 cups) chicken broth
1/4 cup barley
2 tablespoons French lentils
2 medium onions, sliced
4–6 medium carrots, chopped
2 medium parsnips, chopped
1/2 medium rutabaga, chopped
Ground black pepper
2 sprigs of thyme
2 bay leaves
Sprig of parsley
1 pound potatoes in their skins, chopped (about 3 cups)
1 small cabbage, chopped
1 leek, chopped
1/4 cup chopped fresh parsley
One x 15-ounce can of red kidney beans, drained and rinsed
1/4 cup chopped fresh chives

1 Place the ham in a pot and cover with broth. Bring to a boil, skim any scum, then add the barley and lentils.

2 Bring to a boil, reduce the heat, and simmer for 15 minutes. Add the onions, carrots, parsnips, rutabaga, pepper, thyme, bay leaves, and sprig of parsley. Bring to a boil, reduce the heat, and simmer gently for another 15 minutes.

3 Add the potatoes and cabbage and return to a boil. Simmer until they are just tender (about 15 minutes).

4 Add the chopped leek and parsley and cook for another 5 minutes or until the leek is just tender.

5 Add the beans and warm through. Ladle into soup bowls and serve sprinkled with chives.

Per portion: 264 cal., 3g fat, 0.8g sat. fat, 0.97g sodium, 42g carbohydrate

tomato, pasta, and flageolet bean soup

The flageolet is the prince of beans, picked when young and tender. Combined with pasta and whole-grain bread, the G.I. of this soup is extremely low.

SERVES 4

2 teaspoons unsalted butter
1 onion, finely chopped
2 garlic cloves, finely chopped
Large pinch of dried red pepper flakes
One x 14 1/2-ounce can of chopped tomatoes with basil
4 cups vegetable broth
1 cup small pasta shapes
1 sachet bouquet garni (or parsley, thyme, and a bay leaf tied in cheesecloth)
One x 15-ounce can of flageolet beans (canned in water), drained and rinsed
Ground black pepper
2 tablespoons pesto (optional)

1 Melt the butter in a pot, then fry the onion, garlic, and red pepper flakes until soft but still colorless, adding a dash of water if necessary to prevent sticking. Add the tomatoes, broth, pasta, and bouquet garni, and simmer for 15 minutes. Stir in the beans, return to a simmer, and season to taste with black pepper. Add extra broth to thin as necessary.

2 Serve in warm soup bowls, with a little pesto, if you like, and some hot crusty whole-grain bread.

Per portion: 176 cal., 4g fat, 2g sat. fat, 0.54g sodium, 27g carbohydrate

leek and pea soup

Peas lower the G.I. of a dish, but it doesn't matter if you can't find fresh ones—nowadays frozen peas are just as nutritious. Serve with some whole-grain croutons.

SERVES 4–6

2 teaspoons unsalted butter
2 leeks, chopped, washed, and well drained
1 teaspoon fresh thyme leaves
1 garlic clove, finely chopped
4 cups chicken or vegetable broth
10 ounces shelled or frozen peas (about 2^1/$_4$ cups)
1 round lettuce, washed and chopped
1 tablespoon finely chopped mint
Ground black pepper

1 Melt the butter in a pot and cook the leeks with the thyme and garlic over a gentle heat until soft but not brown, adding a dash of water if necessary to prevent sticking.

2 Add the broth and bring to a boil. Add the peas and lettuce and continue cooking until the peas are tender.

3 Stir in the mint and, if you like, blend about half the mixture. Return to the rest of the soup, reheat, and season to taste with black pepper.

Per portion: 101 cal., 5g fat, 2.1g sat. fat, 0.29g sodium, 10g carbohydrate

barley and bean soup

Barley (also called pearl barley) is literally the pearl of the barley as the outer layers, including the bran, have been stripped off and it is then polished until smooth. Even though most of the fiber has been removed, it is still nutritious and a common ingredient in soups.

SERVES 4–6

2 tablespoons olive oil
1 large onion, chopped
2 garlic cloves, chopped
^{3}/$_4$ cup barley or whole-grain barley
1 teaspoon fresh thyme leaves
1 bay leaf
5 cups chicken broth
One x 15-ounce can of black-eyed peas or kidney beans
    (canned in water), drained and rinsed
Ground black pepper
2 tablespoons chopped mint
2 tablespoons chopped cilantro
1 tablespoon chopped chives

1 Heat the oil in a pot and cook the onion and garlic gently until soft but still colorless—this should take about 10 minutes. Add the barley, thyme, and bay leaf, stir to combine. Add the chicken broth and heat to boiling, reduce the heat, and simmer for about 1 hour. Add the beans for the last 10 minutes.

2 Blend half the soup (if you wish) then return to the rest of the soup and season with black pepper. Add extra broth to thin as necessary. Just before serving, stir in the herbs.

Per portion: 274 cal, 7g fat, 1.0g sat. fat, 0.52g sodium, 48g carbohydrate

celtic lamb and barley soup

SERVES 8

Heaped ¹/₂ cup barley or brown whole-grain barley
3 lamb shanks
2 carrots, sliced
2 celery stalks, sliced
1 onion, chopped
2 leeks, shredded and washed
2 bay leaves
2 parsnips, sliced
2 turnips, chopped
Heart of a small cabbage, shredded
2 potatoes with skins, chopped
Ground black pepper
2 tablespoons chopped parsley

1 Cover the barley with cold water, bring to a boil, and strain. Trim the lamb of excess fat and place in a pot with 3 quarts water, the barley, carrots, celery, onions, leeks, and bay leaves. Bring to a boil, skim, reduce the heat, and simmer for 2 hours.

2 Let cool overnight, and remove any fat that forms. Remove the meat and shred into small pieces. Return the meat to the broth and add the remaining vegetables.

3 Cook for another 15 minutes until the vegetables are tender, topping up with more broth as necessary. Season with pepper and serve sprinkled with chopped parsley.

Per portion: 246 cal., 8g fat, 3.5g sat. fat, 0.06g sodium, 29g carbohydrate

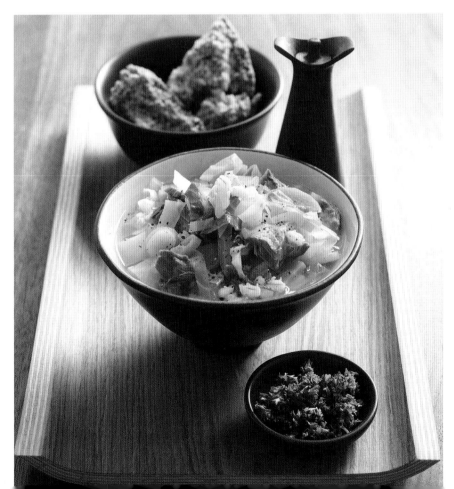

pumpkin and white bean soup

You will never run out of uses for pumpkin. Roast it, mash it, or put it in a pie or soup, and while it is cooking, carve a ghoulish face in the shell.

SERVES 6

1 small pumpkin, peeled, seeded and chopped
2 leeks, white part only, finely sliced
1 carrot, finely chopped
2 stalks of celery, finely chopped
2 garlic cloves, finely chopped
12 fresh sage leaves, shredded
1 tablespoon olive oil
5 cups chicken or vegetable broth
2 bay leaves
One x 15-ounce can of cannellini beans (canned in water), drained and rinsed (if unavailable, use navy or other beans)
2 tablespoons chopped fresh parsley
Ground black pepper
Grated Parmesan, for serving (optional)

1 In a pot, fry the vegetables, garlic, and sage in the olive oil, and cook for about 7 minutes, adding a dash of water to prevent sticking.

2 Pour in the broth and bay leaves and bring to a boil. Reduce the heat and simmer for 15–20 minutes. Add the beans, heat through, then stir in the parsley. Season with black pepper to taste.

3 Serve as a chunky soup (or if preferred, puree half and return to the rest of the soup). Sprinkle with Parmesan, if desired, and eat with whole-grain bread.

Per portion: 124 cal., 4g fat, 0.6g sat. fat, 0.20g sodium, 16g carbohydrate

chicken, chile and corn soup

This is a classic Mexican recipe and a really comforting dish. If you like, you can thicken the broth by mixing 1–2 teaspoons of cornstarch with a little of the broth before adding the rest.

SERVES 4–6

1 teaspoon unsalted butter
4 jalapeño (medium-strength) chiles, seeded and finely chopped
2 slices back bacon (Canadian bacon), chopped
1 onion, finely chopped
1 garlic clove, finely chopped
1 teaspoon fresh thyme leaves
1 large sweet potato, peeled and chopped
2 skinless chicken breast fillets, chopped
1 cup fresh, frozen, or canned corn kernels
5 cups chicken broth
Ground black pepper

1 Melt the butter in a nonstick pot and fry the chiles, bacon, onion, and garlic until the onion is soft, adding a dash of water if necessary to prevent sticking.

2 Add the remaining ingredients and simmer, covered, for 20 minutes. Season to taste with black pepper.

Per portion: 141 cal., 3g fat, 1.2g sat. fat, 0.57g sodium, 11g carbohydrate

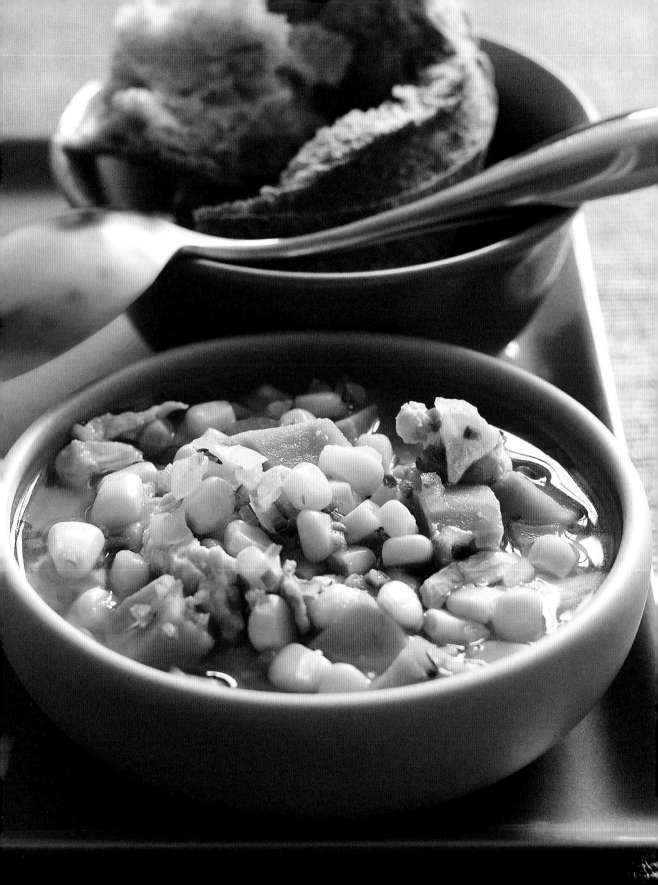

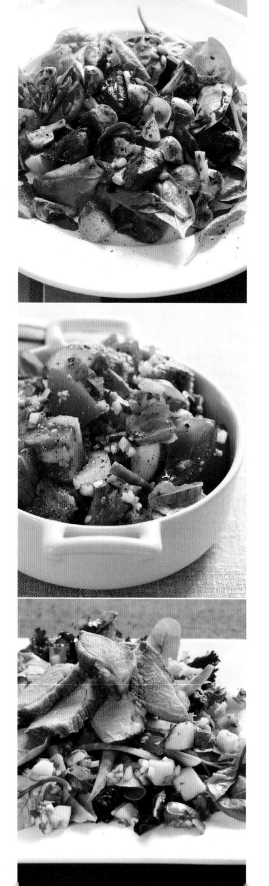

salads

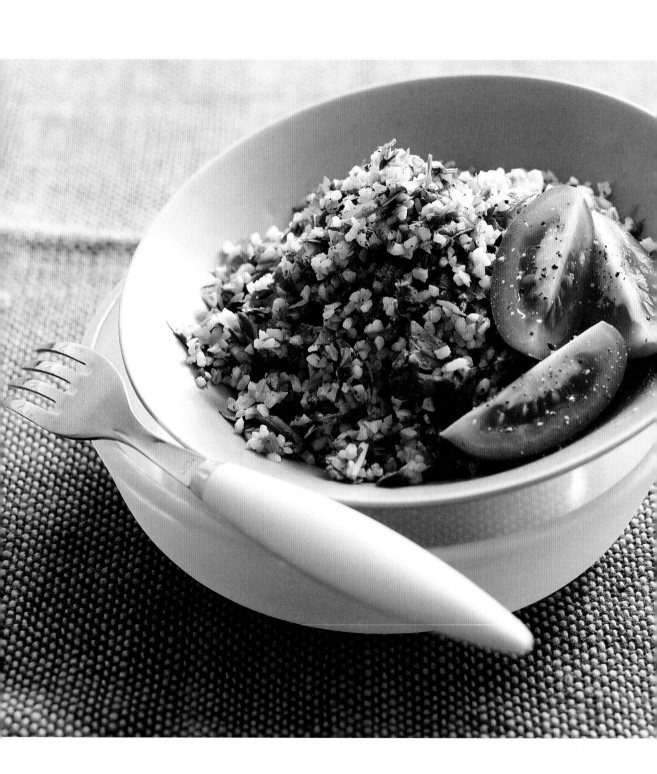

tabbouleh

A classic Middle Eastern salad, this makes a perfect appetizer or accompaniment to the kofta meatballs on page 134. Or make a mezze with falafel (page 82), or either of the eggplant recipes on pages 84–85, together with radishes, lettuce leaves, and whole-wheat flatbread and finish off with mint tea.

SERVES 4

1 cup cracked wheat
Salt and ground black pepper
Juice of 2 small lemons
2 tablespoons extra-virgin olive oil
3 ounces flat-leaf parsley, chopped (about 1 1/2 cups)
1 ounce (about 2 handfuls) mint leaves, chopped
Bunch of scallions, finely sliced
3 plum tomatoes, quartered

1 Soak the cracked wheat in cold water for 20 minutes, drain, and squeeze dry. Put the wheat in a glass bowl, season with salt and black pepper, and add the lemon juice and the olive oil. Let it rest for 30 minutes.

2 Add the parsley, mint, and scallions. Check the seasoning and top the salad with the plum tomatoes.

Per portion: 227 cal., 7g fat, 0.9g sat. fat, 0.21g sodium, 37g carbohydrate

herbed leaf salad

There are two ways of seasoning a salad. You can either season the dressing or the salad itself, but this can lead to trouble because if you season the greens themselves and the greens are damp, you're likely to end up with a mouthful of salt. The way around this is to season around the inside of the bowl (before dressing the salad) and toss the greens in the bowl. In theory they will then be evenly seasoned.

SERVES 4–6

1 garlic clove, peeled
1/4 cup mixed fresh herbs, washed and dried
    (chervil, tarragon, dill, basil, marjoram, flat-leaf parsley,
    mint, chives, or sorrel)
12 ounces mixed salad greens, washed, dried, and torn—
    about 10–12 cups (curly chicory, baby spinach, arugula,
    radicchio, Belgian endive, watercress, trevise, oak leaf,
    dandelion, nasturtium)
Salt and ground black pepper
4–6 tablespoons reduced-calorie salad dressing

1 Rub a wooden salad bowl with the raw garlic. Combine the herbs and the salad greens and mix thoroughly. Season (see above).

2 Dress the salad greens, but don't drown them. Serve immediately—once dressed, try not to let the salad sit around for too long or the leaves will go soggy. If you like, scatter some whole-grain croutons or flakes of Parmesan or pecorino cheese over it.

Per portion: 36 cal., 1.1g fat, 0.1g sat. fat, 0.32g sodium, 5g carbohydrate

salad of asparagus with avocado and walnuts

This is a fusion of Western ingredients with an Eastern dressing. Try to find locally grown asparagus as it will be much more tender and delicious than imported varieties. The asparagus season starts in May, so buy some as soon as it appears in the stores.

SERVES 4

24 asparagus spears, trimmed
1 ripe Hass avocado, pit removed, peeled, and sliced
2 tablespoons lemon juice
2 heads Belgian endive
3 1/2-ounces corn salad (mâche) or watercress, washed
  (about 3 cups)
2 tablespoons walnut pieces
2 tablespoons chopped chives

Dressing
2 tablespoons light soy sauce
1/2 tablespoon grated ginger root
1 garlic clove, crushed
1 tablespoon olive oil
Ground black pepper

1 Cook the asparagus in fast-boiling water for about 5 minutes until just tender, drain and refresh in iced water, drain again, and set aside.

2 Toss the avocado with half the lemon juice.

3 For the dressing, combine the soy, ginger, garlic, remaining lemon juice, and oil, then season with pepper.

4 Arrange the salad greenss on each of four plates, arrange the asparagus spears on top of the greens and drizzle with dressing. Scatter with the walnuts, avocado, and chives.

Per portion without dressing: 141 cal., 11g fat, 1.9g sat. fat, 0.01g sodium, 5g carbohydrate
Per portion with dressing: 172 cal., 13g fat, 2.3g sat. fat, 0.01g sodium, 6g carbohydrate

panzanella

An Italian bread salad, this is one instance where the bread shouldn't be fresh. The base ingredients are bread, tomatoes, and onion, and a handful of fresh basil with a drop or two of olive oil are always welcome.

SERVES 4

2 thick slices day-old whole-grain bread
6 ripe tomatoes, cubed
1 small red onion, finely chopped
1/2 cucumber, chopped
1 stalk of celery, finely sliced
2 garlic cloves, crushed
Small handful of basil leaves, torn into small pieces
2 tablespoons olive oil
1 tablespoon red wine vinegar
Ground black pepper

1 Cut or tear the bread into small pieces.

2 Place the pieces in a bowl and sprinkle with a little cold water—the bread should be moist but not soggy.

3 Add the tomatoes, onion, cucumber, celery, garlic, and basil and mix gently.

4 Mix together the oil and vinegar and season with black pepper. Shake well to make a dressing and pour it over the salad.

5 Toss the salad well, and let it sit for 30 minutes before serving to allow the flavors to develop.

Per portion: 142 cal., 7g fat, 1.1g sat. fat, 0.17g sodium, 17g carbohydrate

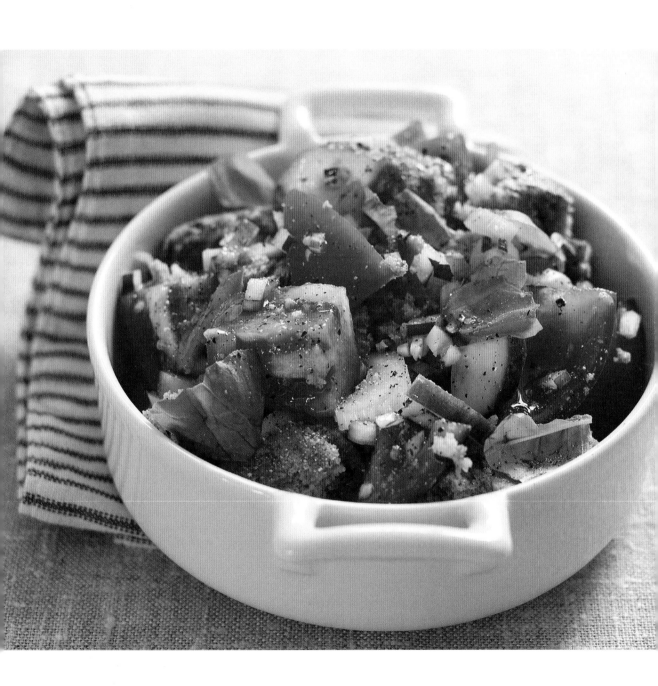

charbroiled vegetable salad

SERVES 4

Olive oil
1 large eggplant, sliced lengthwise
2 large zucchinis, sliced lengthwise
8 scallions, blanched for 2 minutes
1 red pepper, roasted, skinned, seeded and cut into quarters
1 yellow pepper, roasted, skinned, seeded and cut into quarters
12 asparagus spears

Grilled vegetable marinade
1 shallot, chopped
1 red chile, seeded and finely chopped
2 garlic cloves, chopped

8 basil leaves, torn
2 tablespoons extra-virgin olive oil
1 tablespoon sherry vinegar (if unavailable, use red
  wine vinegar)

1 Heat a nonstick ridged grill pan and brush lightly with oil. Cook the vegetables on both sides until cooked to your liking.

2 Combine the marinade ingredients in a bowl or dish and marinate the vegetables overnight. Serve at room temperature.

Per portion: 135 cal., 8g fat, 1.1g sat. fat, 0.09g sodium, 12g carbohydrate

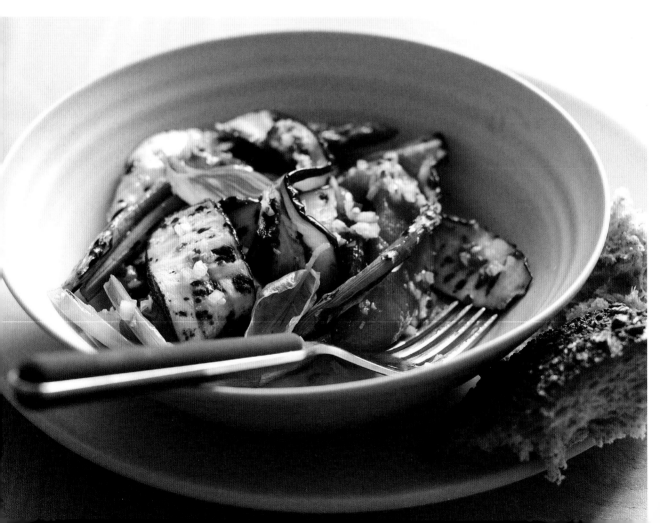

charbroiled radicchio with parmesan shavings

Radicchio is a slightly bitter-tasting red leafy vegetable. As it contains lots of carbs (as well as potassium and magnesium), it is the perfect G.I. addition to a salad.

SERVES 2

2 tablespoons extra-virgin olive oil
1 tablespoon sherry vinegar (if unavailable, use red
   wine vinegar)
2 garlic cloves, crushed
Ground black pepper
1 large head radicchio, quartered
1 lemon, cut in half
1 ounce Parmesan, in 1 piece, shaved into long, thin strips
   using a potato peeler (about 1/2 cup)

1 Heat a ridged grill pan or prepare the barbecue, letting the coals burn down.

2 Combine the oil, vinegar, garlic, and black pepper in a bowl. Marinate the radicchio in this mixture for 5 minutes. Drain, then grill the radicchio for 2 minutes on each side.

3 Serve the radicchio with the lemon halves and a scattering of Parmesan shavings.

Per portion: 183 cal., 16g fat, 4.3g sat. fat, 0.14g sodium, 3g carbohydrate

arugula, belgian endive and parmesan salad

Chicory is part of the same family as radicchio, curly chicory, and witloof (Belgian endive). It is similarly slightly bitter in taste, but this is offset by the lemon and olive oil to make a fresh, zingy salad.

SERVES 2

2 handfuls of arugula, washed and dried
1 head Belgian endive, split into leaves
Ground black pepper
1 tablespoon extra-virgin olive oil
1 ounce good Parmesan (Parmigiano Reggiano), shaved
   into curls with a vegetable peeler (about 1/2 cup)
2 lemon wedges

1 Place the arugula in a salad bowl. Tear the Belgian endive into small pieces and throw in with the arugula.

2 Sprinkle the sides of the bowl with ground black pepper (so that the seasoning doesn't just cling to the greens on top, but coats the greens all over when the salad is tossed). Lightly drizzle olive oil over the salad and toss gently.

3 Scatter Parmesan flakes on top and serve with the lemon, for squeezing over the salad.

Per portion: 127 cal., 10g fat, 3.4g sat. fat, 0.14g sodium, 3g carbohydrate

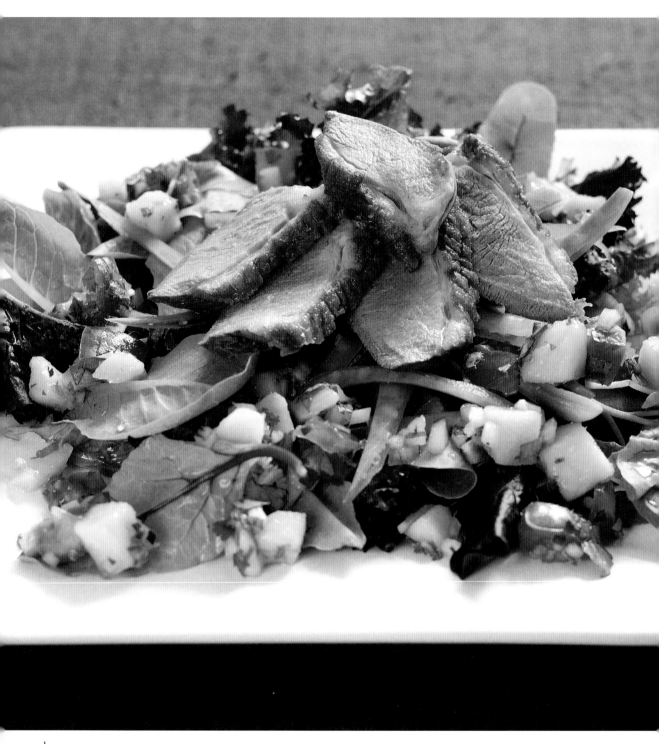

salad of mushrooms, jumbo shrimp & spinach

SERVES 4

One x 8-ounce package button mushrooms, wiped and sliced
6 ounces cooked jumbo shrimp, peeled and cut in half
    (about 1–1 1/2 cups)
5 ounces baby spinach (or other light salad greens—about
    4 1/2–5 cups), washed and dried
2 tablespoons rice vinegar
2 tablespoons lemon juice
1 tablespoon light soy sauce
2 tablespoons vegetable oil
3 scallions, sliced

1 Combine together the mushrooms, shrimp and spinach.

2 In a separate bowl mix the rice vinegar, lemon juice, soy sauce, and vegetable oil. Pour this dressing over the salad, toss well, and sprinkle with the scallions.

Per portion: 124 cal., 7g fat, 0.9g sat. fat, 1.74g sodium, 2g carbohydrate

warm broccoli salad

SERVES 2

1 small onion, grated
4 anchovy fillets, mashed
2 teaspoons capers, rinsed and chopped
Juice of 1/2 small lemon
1 tablespoon extra-virgin olive oil
1 tablespoon chopped mint
10 ounces small broccoli florets (about 5 cups)
Ground black pepper

Thoroughly mix the onion, anchovies, capers, lemon juice, olive oil, and mint in a bowl. Steam the broccoli for 3–5 minutes, then drain and toss with the rest of the salad. Season with black pepper and serve immediately. This salad is also good served at room temperature and is delicious tossed with whole-wheat pasta.

Per portion: 166 cal., 11g fat, 1.1g sat. fat, 0.80g sodium, 6g carbohydrate

duck salad with chunky mango salsa

SERVES 4

2 duck breast fillets, skin on
7 ounces assorted salad greens (about 5 1/2–6 1/2 cups)
4 ounces snow peas (about a handful), shredded, or fine
    green beans, cooked

Salsa
1 mango, pitted, peeled, and chopped
Small bunch of mint, chopped
Small bunch of cilantro, chopped
Juice of 1 lime
1 red onion, chopped
1 chile, seeded and finely chopped
3 tomatoes, chopped
Salt and ground black pepper

1 Preheat the oven to 375°F.

2 Score crisscrosses close together on the skin of the duck; so that most of the fat is released when cooking.

3 Place the duck, skin side down, in an ovenproof frying pan over medium heat and cook for 4–5 minutes. Turn the duck over and cook for 1–2 minutes, then transfer to the oven and cook for 5–10 minutes depending upon how pink you like it.

4 Meanwhile combine the ingredients for the salsa and season. When the duck is cooked, it will feel slightly springy to the touch (if pink) or firm (well done). Remove from the oven and let it rest for 5–10 minutes, then slice. Arrange on the salad greens with the snow peas and serve with the salsa.

Per portion: 151 cal., 5g fat, 1.4g sat. fat, 0.28g sodium, 13g carbohydrate

tuna and bean salad

An all–time favorite Italian salad, this won't take long to make and is great for lunch.

SERVES 2

One x 15-ounce can of cannellini beans, drained and rinsed (if unavailable, use navy or Great Northern beans)
1 small red onion, cut in half and finely sliced
One x 6¹/4-ounce can of good tuna in oil
2 tablespoons roughly chopped flat-leaf parsley
Lemon juice or wine vinegar, to taste
Ground black pepper

Mix all the ingredients together and serve.

Per portion: 328 cal., 10g fat, 1.6g sat. fat, 0.28g sodium, 23g carbohydrate

sardine and potato salad

SERVES 2

9 ounces waxy new potatoes in their skins
One x 3³/4-ounce can of sardines in oil
1 tablespoon lemon juice or wine vinegar, or to taste
1 teaspoon Dijon mustard
Ground black pepper
2 large handfuls of salad greens
3 scallions, finely sliced

1 Steam the potatoes until tender, then slice. While the potatoes are cooking, whisk together the oil from the sardines, lemon juice, and mustard and season with pepper. Thin with a little potato water if you like.

2 Mix the potatoes with the dressing and pile onto the salad greens. Top with the sardines and sprinkle with the scallions and more pepper.

Per portion: 231 cal., 9g fat, 1.9g sat. fat, 0.35g sodium, 22g carbohydrate

warm calf's liver salad

Calf's liver has a soft texture and gentle flavor and is my favorite kind of liver. Although it has fallen out of fashion, liver is a good source of iron, zinc, vitamins A and B₁₂, and protein, but try to buy organic meat.

SERVES 4

6 ounces baby spinach leaves (about 5–6 cups)
2 teaspoons unsalted butter
1 tablespoon olive oil
4 shallots, cut in quarters
1 teaspoon fresh thyme leaves
2 slices back bacon (Canadian bacon), cut in strips
12 ounces calf's, lamb's or chicken livers (about 1¹/2 cups)
24 button mushrooms, quartered
Ground black pepper
2 tablespoons pine nuts
2 tablespoons balsamic vinegar

1 Wash and dry the baby spinach leaves and arrange on four plates.

2 Heat the butter and olive oil in a large nonstick frying pan and fry the shallots until brown and softening. Add the thyme, bacon, and liver, and increase the heat. Cook the liver until brown on all sides but still pink in the middle.

3 Remove liver, shallots, and bacon and keep warm. Add the mushrooms to the pan and toss together, then season with black pepper. With a slotted spoon, place an equal amount on each plate.

4 Add the pine nuts to the pan, and cook until golden, then sprinkle over the salads. Deglaze the pan with the vinegar (ie., heat the vinegar and stir to loosen any bits stuck to the pan) and spoon a little of this warm dressing over each salad.

Per portion: 222 cal., 14g fat, 3.9g sat. fat, 0.33g sodium, 2g carbohydrate

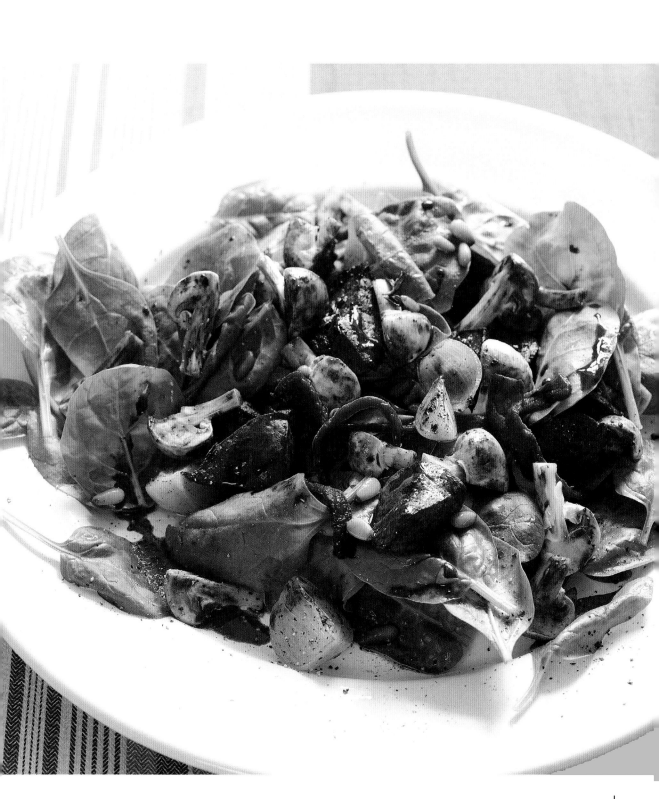

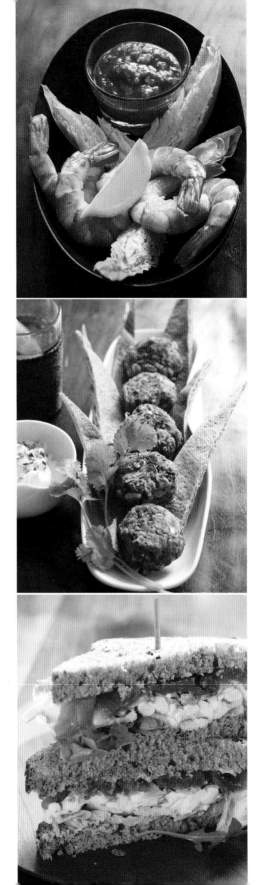

appetizers, sandwiches, and snacks

falafel

A Middle Eastern specialty, falafel is sometimes made with dried fava beans instead of chickpeas, especially in Egypt. A good falafel is light, fragrant, and fluffy with a crisp shell. It is also traditionally deep fried, but this is a much healthier version.

SERVES 4–6—MAKES 24

9 ounces dried chickpeas (about 1²/₃ cups),
    soaked overnight then well drained
1 garlic clove
Handful of parsley
Handful of cilantro
2 tablespoons chopped mint
¹/₂ onion, roughly chopped
¹/₄ teaspoon cayenne pepper
¹/₂ teaspoon ground cumin
¹/₂ teaspoon ground black pepper
¹/₂ teaspoon baking powder
¹/₂ teaspoon ground coriander
Vegetable oil for frying
Low-fat plain yogurt, or whole-wheat pita, shredded salad
    greens and pickled chiles for serving (optional)

1 Blend all the ingredients except the last two in a food processor to form a manageable mixture.

2 Shape into 24 small patties and fry in a thin film of oil in a nonstick frying pan until golden brown on both sides. Serve as a snack with plain yogurt—or for a more substantial meal, in pita bread pockets with shredded salad greens and pickled chiles.

Per portion: 135 cal., 7g fat, 0.7g sat. fat, 0.06g sodium, 13g carbohydrate

piquant avocado salsa

Avocados are full of heart-protective monounsaturates. Their sweet, creamy flavor is tempered here by the herbs and spices to make a great appetizer or party food.

SERVES 2

1 ripe avocado, peeled and pitted
1 tomato, seeded and chopped
2 scallions, sliced
Juice of ¹/₂–1 lime
1 chile, seeded and finely chopped
Pinch of ground cumin
Pinch of ground coriander
2 tablespoons finely chopped cilantro
1 teaspoon chile oil
Salt and ground black pepper

1 Mash the avocado with the back of a fork, but do not make it too smooth. Fold in all the other ingredients and season to taste.

2 Serve with crostini or corn chips.

Per portion: 163 cal., 16g fat, 3.2g sat. fat, 0.21g sodium, 3g carbohydrate

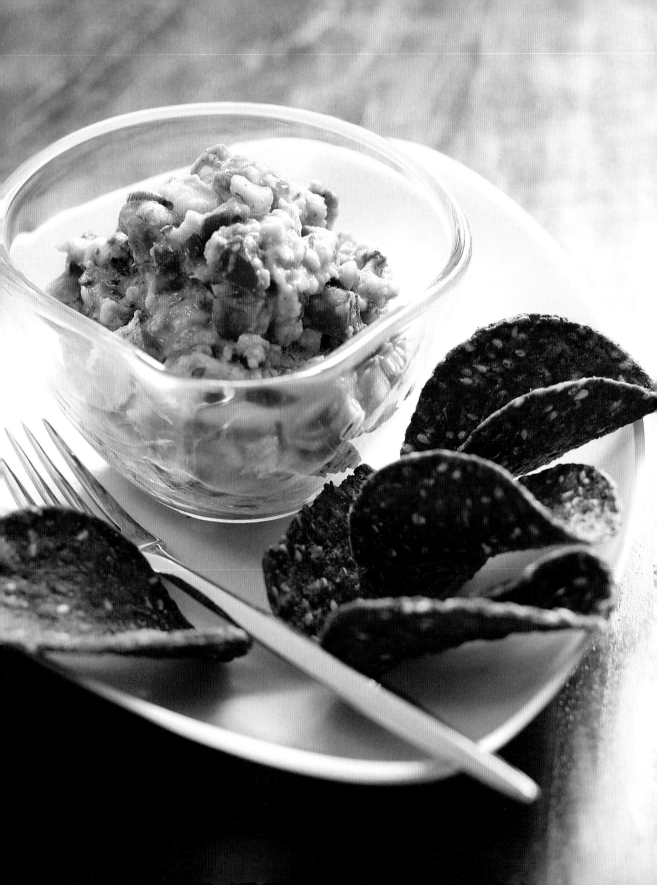

lentil spread

Like tapenade, this Mediterranean paste is made with olives and capers and will keep for 2–3 days if stored in an airtight container and refrigerated. Serve with crostini or bruschetta.

SERVES 6

9 ounces (about 1 1/3 cups) French or European (green) lentils, rinsed
1 1/4 cups vegetable broth
2 tablespoons chopped garlic
2 tablespoons chopped sun-dried tomatoes
1 tablespoon chopped sun-dried peppers (if unavailable, use roasted peeled peppers)
2 tablespoons capers
3 anchovy fillets
3 tablespoons chopped black or green olives
1 tablespoon extra-virgin olive oil
2 tablespoons lemon juice
1/4 cup chopped parsley

1 Cook the lentils in the broth with the garlic, tomatoes, and peppers until just tender—about 20 minutes—adding a little extra broth if necessary to prevent sticking.

2 Put the contents of the pan in a food processor and blend briefly with the rest of the ingredients to make a coarse spread. Add extra broth to soften the mixture as required.

Per portion: 187 cal., 6g fat, 0.6g sat. fat, 0.55g sodium, 24g carbohydrate

eggplant "caviar"

This is a feisty dip with loads of flavor. Eggplants are a good source of fiber and potassium, while the onion, garlic, and ginger will boost your immune system.

SERVES 6

3 large eggplants
1 tablespoon sesame oil
1 small red onion, finely chopped
2 garlic cloves, finely chopped
1 large knob of ginger, peeled and grated
1 red chile, seeded and finely chopped
1 red pepper, roasted or broiled, peeled, seeded and chopped
2–4 scallions, finely sliced
2 tablespoons finely chopped cilantro

1 Preheat the oven to 375°F. Prick the eggplants all over with a fork and bake on a tray for 45–60 minutes or until they feel very soft. Keep warm.

2 Meanwhile, heat the sesame oil in a small frying pan and cook the red onion, garlic, ginger, and chile until soft but not brown.

3 Cut the eggplants in half lengthwise and scoop out the flesh (squeezing out the excess liquid) into a food processor then add the cooked onion mixture. Blend briefly. Fold in the other ingredients. Alternatively, chop the eggplant pulp and stir in the rest of the ingredients.

5 Serve at room temperature with whole-grain toast.

Per portion: 81 cal., 4g fat, 0.7g sat. fat, 0.01g sodium, 10g carbohydrate

chunky eggplant and yogurt dip

Eggplants used to be sliced and covered in salt before cooking to get rid of any bitterness. This is no longer necessary because of revised growing techniques, but it will reduce the amount of oil the eggplant soaks up.

SERVES 4

18 ounces eggplants, cut in 2-inch cubes
1 tablespoon extra-virgin olive oil
18 ounces plum tomatoes, peeled, seeded and cubed
  (about 2 cups)
3/4 cup tomato juice
2 green chiles, finely chopped
1 tablespoon chopped garlic
2 tablespoons white wine vinegar
Salt and ground black pepper
3/4 cup fat-free plain yogurt
4 scallions, finely sliced
2 tablespoons chopped fresh parsley

1 Place the eggplant in a heavy pot along with the olive oil, tomatoes, tomato juice, and chiles. Cook over medium heat for 20 minutes.

2 Stir in the garlic and vinegar and continue to cook for another 20 minutes, adding a little extra tomato juice if necessary until the eggplant is very tender. Season. Remove from the heat, then stir in the yogurt and sprinkle with the scallions and parsley.

3 Serve warm or at room temperature with whole-wheat pita bread or as a vegetable accompaniment.

Per portion: 101 cal., 4g fat, 0.9g sat. fat, 0.35g sodium, 12g carbohydrate

spicy mushrooms on toast

SERVES 2

1 onion, finely chopped
1 teaspoon grated ginger
1 garlic clove, finely chopped
1 chile, seeded and finely chopped
1 tablespoon sesame oil
10 ounces (about 2 1/2–3 cups) button mushrooms, quartered
2/3 cup dry white wine
1 tablespoon light soy sauce
Ground black pepper
2 large slices whole-grain bread, toasted
2 scallions, sliced
1 tablespoon chopped cilantro
1 tablespoon chopped fresh mint
2 tablespoons fat-free plain yogurt

1 Cook the onion, ginger, garlic and chile in the oil over medium heat until the onion is softened. Turn up the heat, add the mushrooms, and cook for 5 minutes.

2 Add the wine and soy sauce and cook for 5 minutes or until the mushrooms are cooked and the liquid has reduced to about 1/4 cup. Season to taste with black pepper.

3 With a slotted spoon, remove the mushrooms and place them on the toast, scatter with the scallions, cilantro and mint, and top with a spoonful of yogurt.

Per portion: 296 cal., 8g fat, 1.3g sat. fat, 0.64g sodium, 33g carbohydrate

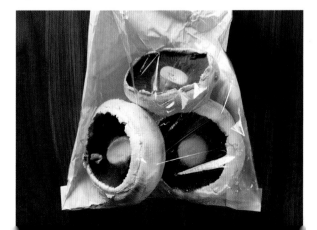

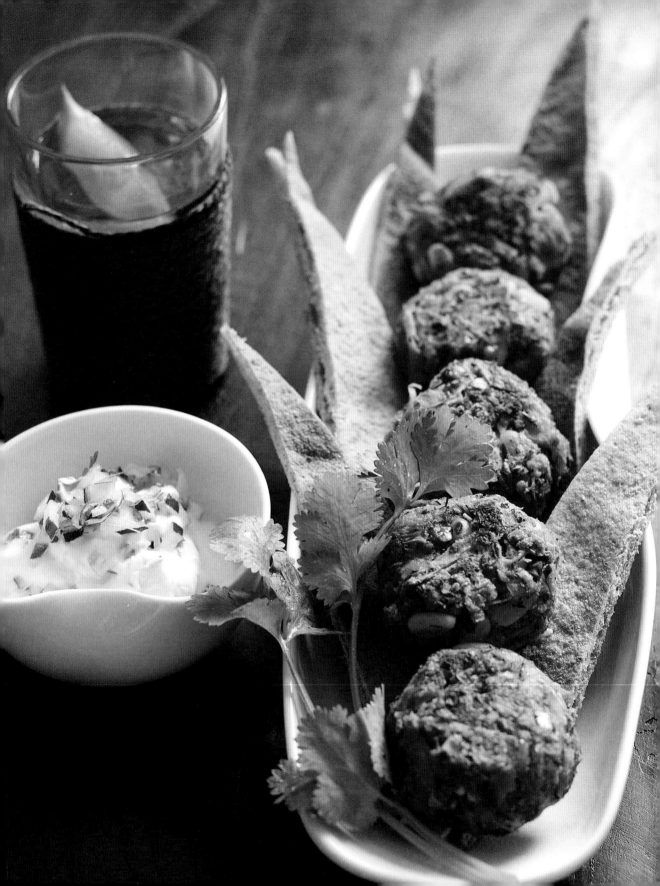

mediterranean carrot mezza

This is a gorgeous mix of carrots, fruit, nuts, and spices. Make them in advance and take them as a packed lunch.

SERVES 4—MAKES 24

10 medium carrots
2 slices whole-grain bread, rubbed into crumbs
12 dried apricots, finely chopped
1 tablespoon golden raisins, chopped
4 scallions, finely chopped
3 tablespoons pine nuts
1 teaspoon red pepper flakes
2 teaspoons finely grated orange zest
1 egg
6 tablespoons mixed chopped fresh mint and dill
Salt and ground black pepper
Sunflower oil for frying

For serving
Low-fat plain yogurt
Chopped red onion
Cilantro leaves, shredded

1 Steam and roughly mash half the carrots, and grate the rest. Combine them together then add the remaining ingredients up to the seasoning and knead well. If the mixture is too wet, add more bread crumbs—it should be soft and slightly damp.

2 Mold the mixture into 24 small "cakes" then "dry" fry in a nonstick pan sprayed with oil until browned on both sides.

3 Serve with low-fat plain yogurt, generously flavored with red onion and cilantro.

Per portion: 264 cal., 10g fat, 1.2g sat. fat, 0.39g sodium, 40g carbohydrate

fava bean and rosemary mash

Great as a vegetable with grilled meats or fish, you could also serve this as a dip with bruschetta or whole-wheat pita bread. If you prefer, you could choose other beans or peas.

SERVES 6

1 tablespoon extra-virgin olive oil
2 garlic cloves, crushed
1 tablespoon very finely chopped fresh rosemary (if using peas, use 1–2 tablespoons mint instead)
1 small onion, finely chopped
1 pound cooked fava beans, with some cooking liquor (about 3^1/$_2$ cups)
Juice of ^{1}/$_2$ lemon
Ground black pepper

1 Pour the olive oil into a pan then add the garlic, rosemary, and onion and cook over medium heat until the onion is soft but still colorless.

2 Add the beans, lemon juice, and a generous grinding of pepper and cook gently for 10 minutes. Remove from the heat and roughly mash or blend in a food processor. Add some bean cooking liquor if the mixture is too dry.

Per portion: 87 cal., 4g fat, 0.5g sat. fat, 0.02g sodium, 8g carbohydrate

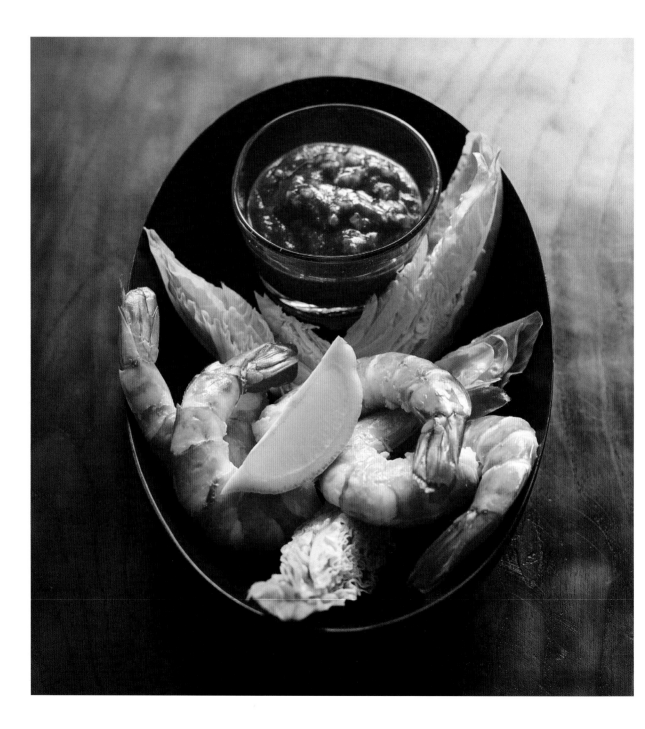

american shrimp cocktail

The American shrimp cocktail is very different from the British prawn cocktail. Americans use large cooked shrimp and serve it with a hot red cocktail sauce whereas in Britain, small shrimp are drowned in mayonnaise, mixed with Worcestershire sauce and ketchup, then sprinkled with paprika.

SERVES 6

1 pound cooked large shrimp (about 30), shelled and deveined
4 Bibb (limestone) lettuces, quartered
Lemon wedges, for serving

Sauce
1/3 cup chili sauce
1/3 cup reduced-sugar and salt ketchup
1/2 tablespoon fresh lemon juice
1 tablespoon grated horseradish (not creamed)
Dash of Worcestershire sauce
1/2 stalk of celery, very finely chopped
Dash of Tabasco sauce

1 Combine all the sauce ingredients and keep in the fridge until needed.

2 Arrange the shrimp on a platter with the lettuce and lemon wedges. Serve the cocktail sauce separately.

Per portion: 99 cal., 1g fat, 0.1g sat. fat, 0.36g sodium, 8g carbohydrate

kipper pâté

A kippered herring is quintessentially British, but the French have claimed that the kipper was first made in the north of France. Either way, I have transformed it into a low-fat pâté that is perfect for a light lunch.

SERVES 4

3 cooked kippered herring fillets, skinned
1/3 cup low-fat cream cheese or cottage cheese
6 tablespoons low-fat plain yogurt
Lemon juice, to taste
Pinch of chili powder
1/2 teaspoon freshly ground black pepper
Pinch of nutmeg

1 Put the cooked kippers in a food processor along with the cheese, yogurt, lemon juice, chili powder, pepper, and nutmeg. Blend until fairly smooth. Season to taste. Transfer to a bowl, cover, and refrigerate overnight.

2 Serve the pâté with hot whole-grain toast and cucumber stalks or cherry tomatoes, if you wish.

Per portion: 176 cal., 11g fat, 2.1g sat. fat, 0.59g sodium, 5g carbohdrate

purple figs with prosciutto and minted yogurt

SERVES 4

Minted yogurt
2 tablespoons finely chopped cucumber
2/3 cup low-fat plain yogurt
1 tablespoon chopped fresh mint
Ground black pepper

8 large ripe purple figs
7 ounces thinly sliced prosciutto (about 12–14 slices)

1 To make the minted yogurt, combine all the ingredients and season to taste with black pepper.

2 Slice the figs vertically into 4 and arrange on plates with the prosciutto. Serve the yogurt separately.

Per portion: 363 cal., 8g fat, 2.3 sat. fat, 1.09g sodium, 56g carbohydrate

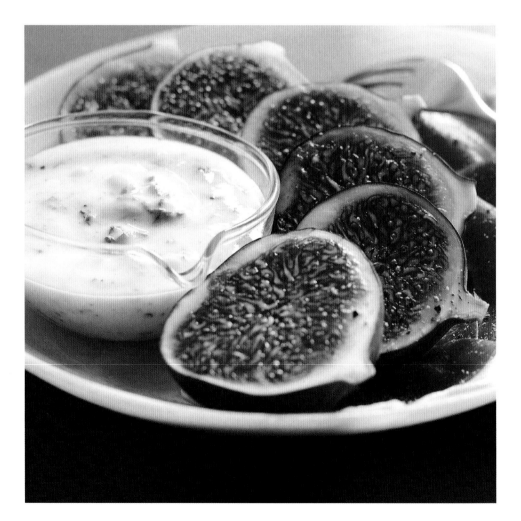

spiced chicken pita sandwich

More of a meal than a snack, this is reminiscent of the Greek souvlaki, aromatic pita bread stuffed with spiced lamb and yogurt.

SERVES 4

2 onions, thinly sliced
2 garlic cloves
$1/2$ teaspoon ground cinnamon
1 teaspoon ground cumin
1 teaspoon ground coriander
2 teaspoons ground paprika
$1/2$ teaspoon chili powder
$1/4$ cup chopped fresh cilantro
2 tablespoons chopped fresh mint
12 ounces chicken stir-fry pieces (about $1 1/2$ cups)
1 tablespoon olive oil
4 whole-wheat pita breads
$1/4$ iceberg lettuce, shredded
Shredded red pepper and cucumber (optional)
$1/4$ cup fat-free plain yogurt

1 Put half the onion, the garlic, the five spices, and half the herbs into a food processor and blend until thick and smooth. Pour into a bowl and combine with the chicken. Let it marinate for 30–60 minutes or overnight.

2 Heat the olive oil in a nonstick frying pan and fry the remaining onion slices until soft. Remove the chicken from the marinade, scraping off the marinade (the more you leave on, the hotter the chicken will be), and add the chicken to the onion. Pan-fry until the chicken is cooked—about 5 minutes.

3 While the chicken is cooking, lightly toast the pita bread on both sides. Split the side of each pita to create a pocket. Put some lettuce in the bottom, fill with the chicken, red pepper, and cucumber (if using), and top with a spoonful of yogurt and a sprinkling of the remaining mint and cilantro.

Per portion: 422 cal., 5g fat, 0.7g sat. fat, 0.55g sodium, 64g carbohydrate

smoked salmon (lox) and cottage cheese sandwich

SERVES 1

2 slices whole-grain bread
Scraping of butter or low-fat spread (optional)
$1/2$ Bibb (limestone) lettuce, separated into leaves
Small handful of arugula
$1/3$ cup low-fat cream cheese or cottage cheese
$1/4$ red onion, finely sliced
1 ounce thinly sliced smoked salmon (lox)—about
   2–3 tablespoons
1 tablespoon capers
Ground black pepper

Spread both slices of bread with a little butter or low-fat spread, if you like. Top one slice with lettuce, arugula, cheese, red onion, smoked salmon, and capers, seasoning with pepper as you layer. Finish with the final slice of bread.

Per portion: 279 cal., 5g fat, 1.3 sat. fat, 1.18g sodium, 38g carbohydrate

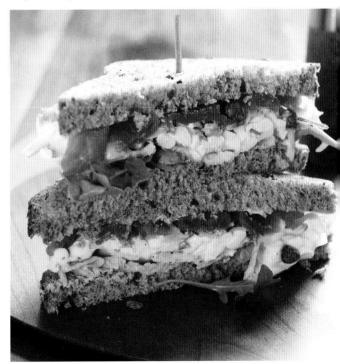

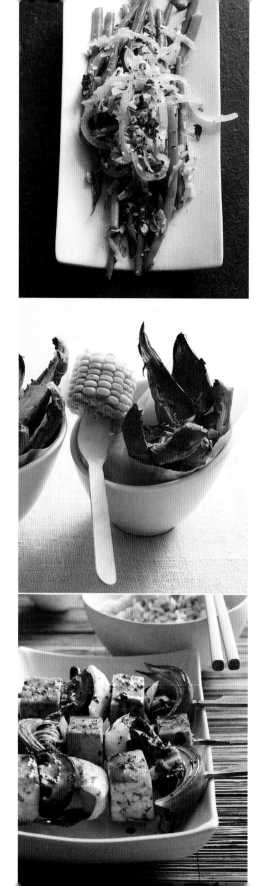

vegetables

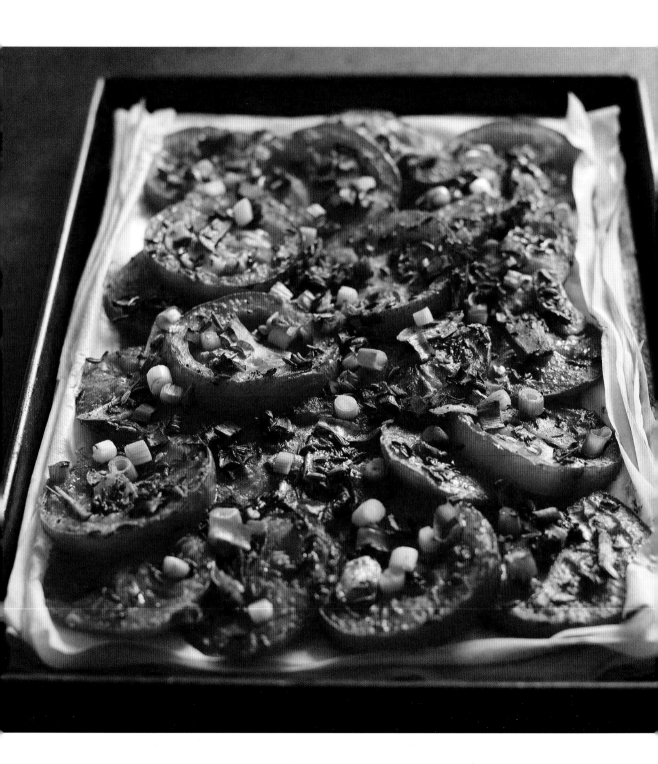

aromatic tomato tart

This exquisite tart is very simple to prepare and can be eaten either alone or as part of a main course. Tomatoes are low-G.I. and full of vitamin C. Cooking tomatoes, especially in olive oil, helps to release lycopene, an antioxidant and the reason why tomatoes are red.

SERVES 4

4 sheets phyllo dough
2 tablespoons olive oil
$1/2$ teaspoon ground coriander
$1/2$ teaspoon fennel seeds
3 scallions, sliced
1 teaspoon cumin seeds
2 garlic cloves, sliced
$1/4$ teaspoon chili powder
6 large ripe tomatoes, each cut into 4 thick slices

1 Preheat the oven and a nonstick baking tray to 425°F.

2 Lightly brush the sheets of phyllo dough with a little of the olive oil and fold them in half. Stack them, one on top of the other, on another nonstick baking tray (one which would fit inside the other baking tray).

3 In a frying pan, warm the rest of the oil over medium heat. Add the ground coriander, fennel seeds, scallions, cumin seeds, and garlic, and stir-fry until the spices start releasing their fragrant bouquet. Add the chili powder and the tomatoes (you will need to do this in two batches), and cook for 1–2 minutes, being careful not to break up the tomato slices. Set aside any cooking juices.

4 Arrange the tomatoes on the dough, leaving a 1/4-inch edge around the dough. Set the baking tray on top of the hot tray in the oven and cook for 15–20 minutes, until the pastry is crisp and golden.

5 Drizzle any tomato spice juices over the tart and serve.

Per portion: 110 cal., 8g fat, 1.6g sat. fat, 0.04g sodium, 9g carbohydrate

barley and goat cheese soufflé bake

Don't be afraid of this as it's more of a light vegetable bake than a true soufflé and it's not the least bit temperamental. Serve with tomato sauce (page 152) and a green salad.

SERVES 4

$2/3$ cup brown whole-grain barley or regular barley
1 tablespoon olive oil
1 medium onion, finely chopped
1 garlic clove, crushed
1 stalk of celery, finely sliced
1 carrot, finely sliced
$1/2$ red pepper, finely chopped
$1/4$ teaspoon dried crushed chilies
3 egg whites
4 ounces goat cheese, crumbled (about 1 cup)
Ground black pepper

1 Bring 1½ cups water to a boil in a medium saucepan. Add the barley and simmer, covered, for 35–40 minutes, or until just tender. Drain and set aside.

2 Preheat the oven to 400°F.

3 Heat the oil in a frying pan over medium heat. Add the onion, cook for 5 minutes, then add the garlic, remaining vegetables and chiles and cook for another 5 minutes.

4 Add the barley to the frying pan and toss with the vegetable mixture. Cook for 5 minutes, stirring occasionally. Transfer to a bowl and let cool.

5 In a large bowl, whisk the egg whites until soft peaks form —the mixture should be stiff, but not dry. Stir a third of the egg whites into the cooled barley mixture. Then fold in the remaining whites. Fold in the goat cheese. Season with black pepper. Spoon the mixture into a buttered shallow ovenproof dish. Bake until golden, about 20 minutes.

Per portion: 226 cal., 8g fat, 3.1g sat. fat, 0.38g sodium, 33g carbohydrate

spaghetti with herby tomato sauce

This is a recipe with huge potential. This traditional sauce can be adapted according to your tastes and content of your cupboard—add capers, olives, or mushrooms, or try replacing the sugar with a small piece of dark chocolate.

SERVES 3

1 tablespoon extra-virgin olive oil
1 small onion, finely chopped
2 garlic cloves, finely chopped
1 stalk of celery, finely chopped
18 ounces tomatoes, peeled and quartered
   (about $2^1/2$–$3^1/2$ cups)
1 teaspoon raw cane sugar
$2/3$ cup red wine
3 tablespoons torn basil leaves
1 tablespoon chopped parsley
9 ounces dried spaghetti
Salt and ground black pepper
1 ounce freshly grated Parmesan (about $1/2$ cup)

1 Heat the olive oil in a medium-sized saucepan and cook the onion, garlic, and celery until soft but not brown. Add the tomatoes, sugar, and red wine.

2 Cook for 20 minutes over medium heat, stirring from time to time. Remove from the heat and stir in the basil and parsley. Meanwhile, cook the spaghetti in plenty of fast-boiling water until al dente. Drain well.

3 Toss the spaghetti with the sauce, season to taste, and top with the Parmesan.

Per portion: 434 cal., 9g fat, 2.4g sat. fat, 0.32g sodium, 71g carbohydrate

spicy beans with carrot and coconut

Influenced by Indian cooking and full of wonderful spices and aromas, this recipe gives beans a much needed wake-up call. Lightly roasting the hazelnuts improves their flavor and if you are a vegetarian, the nuts are a good alternative source of iron. If you are allergic, leave them out and use vegetable oil instead.

SERVES 6–8

18 ounces extra-fine haricot verts (young green beans),
   topped and tailed (about $3^1/2$–$4^1/2$ cups)
2 tablespoons peanut or vegetable oil
1 teaspoon black mustard seeds
1 chile, seeded and finely chopped
2 small onions, finely sliced
2 garlic cloves, finely chopped
2 teaspoons grated ginger
1 teaspoon ground turmeric
$1/4$ teaspoon ground cardamom
4 ounces carrots, coarsely grated (about $3/4$ cup)
$3/4$ cup vegetable broth
$1/2$ cup dry, unsweetened coconut
$1/4$ cup chopped roasted hazelnuts
2 tablespoons chopped cilantro

1 Steam the beans for about 4 minutes until just tender, then set aside.

2 Heat the oil in a frying pan, add the mustard seeds, cover and cook over medium heat until the seeds start to pop. Add the chile, onions, garlic, ginger, turmeric, and cardamom. Cook, stirring, for 4 minutes until the onions start to soften.

3 Add the carrots, broth, and coconut, and cook for 5 minutes.

4 Finally add the beans, hazelnuts, and cilantro and cook for 1–2 minutes to infuse the flavors and warm the beans.

5 Serve with rice or grilled or roast meats or fish.

Per portion: 124 cal., 10g fat, 2.9g sat. fat, 0.20g sodium, 7g carbohydrate

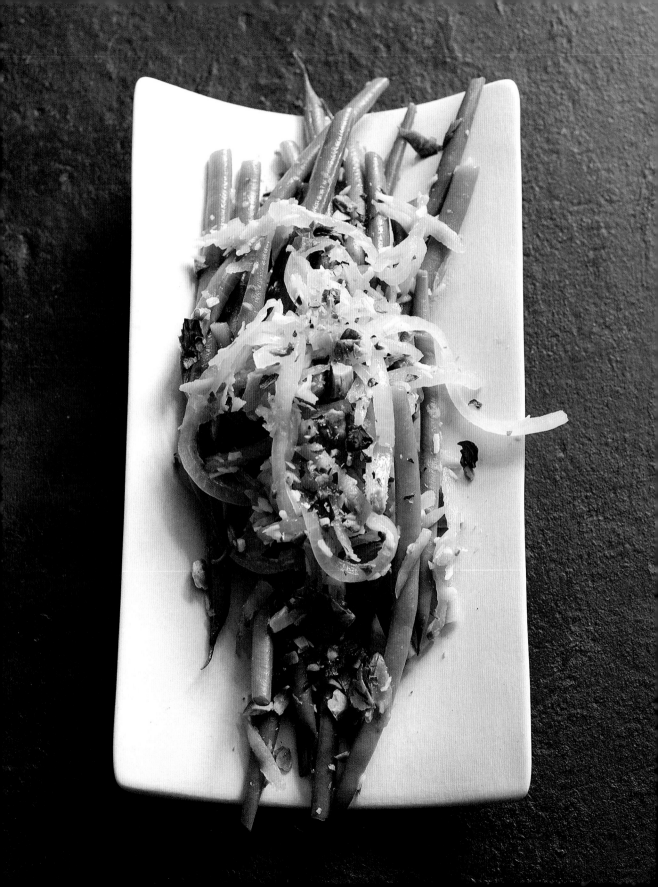

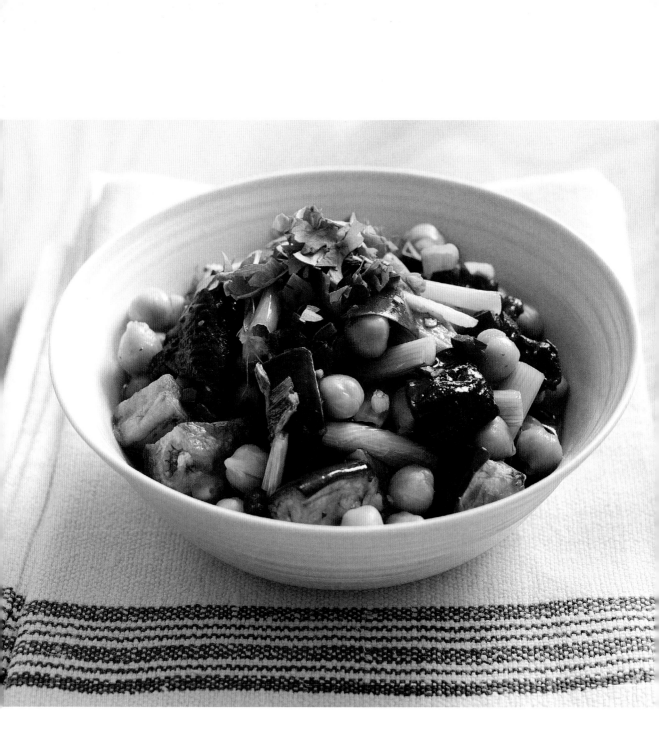

spicy braised eggplants with chickpeas & prunes

The prunes may surprise you but they add a touch of sweetness. Dried fruit is common in Middle Eastern dishes and increases the fiber and lowers the G.I. of a dish. Serve with basmati rice.

SERVES 4

2 large eggplants, cut in 1-inch cubes
1 tablespoon vegetable oil
1 tablespoon sesame oil
1 tablespoon finely chopped garlic
1 tablespoon grated fresh ginger
2 bunches of scallions, cut in 1-inch sticks
One x 15-ounce can of chickpeas, drained and rinsed
1³/4 cup vegetable broth
1 tablespoon light soy sauce
6 ounces ready-to-eat pitted prunes (about 1 cup), cut in half
2 teaspoons cornstarch, mixed to a paste with a little water
2 tablespoons chopped cilantro
1 chile, seeded and finely chopped

1 Toss the eggplant cubes in the vegetable oil in a shallow baking pan and place in a single layer under a preheated broiler until lightly charred—this should take 10–15 minutes and they will need turning and shaking occasionally.

2 Heat the sesame oil in a large wok, then add the garlic, ginger, and scallions and cook for 5 minutes, turning regularly. Add the eggplant to the pan, along with the chickpeas, broth, and soy sauce and bring to a boil.

3 Add the prunes and cook for another 10 minutes. Add the cornstarch and stir to thicken. Pour the mixture into a dish and sprinkle with the cilantro and chile.

Per portion: 223 cal., 8g fat, 1.0g sat. fat, 0.44g sodium, 31g carbohydrate

oriental greens with oyster sauce

Choose "strong" greens such as bok choy, Swiss chard, spinach, or any of the Oriental greens available in Chinese markets. This easy recipe brings out the sweetness of the vegetables in the blanching process while the sauce adds a rich, almost nutty flavor.

SERVES 4

18 ounces Oriental greens, leaves separated and roughly chopped, if you wish (about 8–9 cups)
1 teaspoon sesame oil
1 teaspoon peanut or vegetable oil
¹/2-inch piece of fresh ginger root, peeled and finely grated
1 red chile, seeded and finely chopped
1 garlic clove, finely chopped
2 tablespoons oyster sauce
2 tablespoons Chinese rice wine (mirin) or dry sherry
2 tablespoons light soy sauce
¹/2 tablespoon honey

1 Bring a large pot of water to a rolling boil, add the greens, and blanch for 1–3 minutes, depending upon the vegetable you are using, until wilted and just tender but still with a bite. Drain well and place on a warm serving dish. Keep warm.

2 Meanwhile, heat the sesame and the peanut or vegetable oil in a small frying pan. Add the ginger, chile, and garlic and cook for 2 minutes, stirring, then stir in the oyster sauce, mirin or sherry, soy sauce and honey. Just heat through and drizzle over the greens for serving.

Per portion: 90 cal., 3g fat, 0.4g sat. fat, 0.34g sodium, 9g carbohydrate

grilled vegetable pizza

SERVES 4—MAKES 1 X 14-INCH PIZZA OR 2 X 9-INCH

Whole-grain pizza dough
9 ounces (about 1³/₄–2 cups) whole-grain flour
1 envelope rapid-rise yeast
Pinch of sugar
¹/₂ teaspoon salt
1 tablespoon olive oil

4 plum tomatoes, cut into rough chunks
4 ounces wood-roasted onion, cut in half if large
4 ounces broiled artichokes, (drained and quartered)
4 ounces wood-roasted red peppers, drained and sliced
　(about ²/₃ cup)—if unavailable, then broil the peppers
1 tablespoon oregano leaves
4 ounces ricotta (about ¹/₂ cup)
Small handful of arugula leaves
¹/₄ cup pine nuts, toasted

1 To make the pizza dough, combine the flour, yeast, sugar, salt, olive oil, and about ²/₃ cup hand-hot water, and mix well with a wooden spoon.

2 Turn out onto a counter and knead for 7–10 minutes, until smooth and elastic. The dough should feel moist to the touch. You can use an electric mixer with a dough hook—mix for 5–7 minutes—or a food processor for 1 minute.

3 Place the dough in a lightly oiled bowl and turn to coat the top with oil. Cover with plastic wrap and let it rise in a warm place for 30–60 minutes until doubled in size.

4 Preheat the oven to 425°F. Roll out the pizza base and scatter the vegetables and oregano on top. Dot with ricotta and season with pepper. Bake for about 15 minutes. Scatter with arugula leaves and pine nuts and serve at once.

**Per portion – pizza topping: 137 cal., 8g fat,
2.3g sat. fat, 0.06g sodium, 12g carbohydrate
Per portion – pizza dough: 344 cal., 17g fat,
2.4g sat. fat, 0.25g sodium, 44g carbohydrate**

corn pudding

This also makes a good quiche filling—line a quiche pan or shallow cake pan with very thinly rolled out whole-grain bread dough (see recipe, left) and bake as below.

SERVES 6

2 teaspoons unsalted butter
1 small onion, finely chopped
1 garlic clove, finely chopped
1 teaspoon fresh thyme leaves
¹/₂ green pepper, finely chopped
2 green chiles, seeded and finely chopped
Corn kernels from 3 ears of corn or 9 ounces frozen or
　canned corn, about 1 cup, thawed and well drained
¹/₂ teaspoon each of ground black pepper and ground nutmeg
Pinch of cayenne pepper
2 tablespoons cornstarch
1³/₄ cups 2% or low-fat milk
3 eggs
2 tablespoons chopped flat-leaf parsley
1 tablespoon chopped fresh chives
2 ounces freshly grated Parmesan (about 1 cup)
2 ounces Gruyère or Swiss cheese, grated (about ¹/₂ cup)

1 Preheat the oven to 350°F.

2 Heat the butter in a frying pan, add the onion, garlic, thyme, green pepper, and chiles. Cook over medium heat for 3 minutes. Add half the corn and cook for another 5 minutes (2–3, if using frozen or canned). Set aside, then season with pepper, nutmeg, and cayenne.

3 Place the remaining corn in a blender with the cornstarch, milk, and eggs, and blend until smooth. Fold in the corn mixture, herbs, and both cheeses.

4 Pour into a baking dish, place in a hot water bath, and cook until firm, about 1 hour. Let it stand for 10 minutes before serving. Eat as it is or serve cold with meats and salad.

**Per portion: 237 cal., 13g fat, 6.5g sat. fat,
0.23g sodium, 18g carbohydrate**

dal with added spice

Lentils are naturally rich in protein. The body deals efficiently with protein found in meat, fish, and dairy products but the vegetable proteins found in lentils require more effort to digest, so the Indians added certain digestion-friendly spices such as ginger and asafetida. Serve with flatbread or basmati rice.

SERVES 4–6

1^1/$_3$ cups red lentils, washed
2 tablespoons ghee or clarified butter
5 garlic cloves, finely chopped
1 onion, finely chopped
1-inch piece of ginger, peeled and finely chopped
3 green chiles, seeded and finely chopped
1 teaspoon ground coriander
1 teaspoon ground cumin
^{1}/$_2$ teaspoon chili powder
1 teaspoon black mustard seeds
1 teaspoon turmeric
Pinch of asafetida (optional)
3 plum tomatoes, seeded and chopped
3 tablespoons chopped cilantro
2 tablespoons lime juice

1 Pour 2^1/$_2$ cups water into a saucepan over medium heat, add the lentils, and cook for 15 minutes, stirring regularly at first as it is during the early period of cooking that the lentils will stick together.

2 Meanwhile, heat the ghee in a frying pan and add the garlic, onion, ginger, and chiles and cook for 10 minutes over medium heat until the onion has softened. Add the spices and cook for another 2 minutes. Fold into the lentils.

3 Cook the dal for 10–15 minutes, adding a little boiling water if necessary until the lentils are tender and the mixture is slightly sloppy. Fold in the tomatoes, cilantro and lime juice.

Per portion: 286 cal., 8g fat, 4.3g sat. fat, 0.03g sodium, 41g carbohydrate

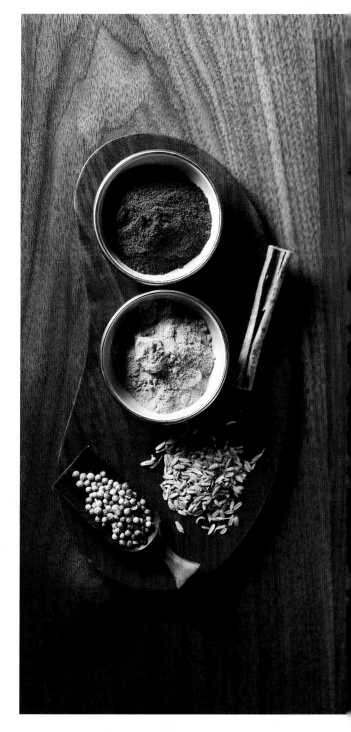

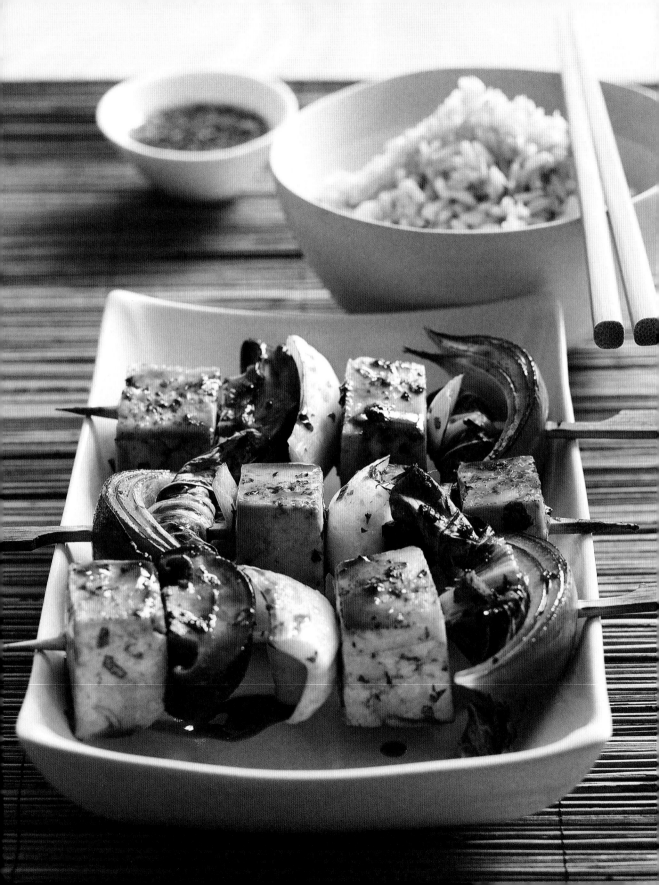

oriental tofu, onion, and mushroom kabobs

These are great kabobs for the barbecue or broiler. Tofu is fermented soybean curd, which not only contains protein but is also full of beneficial phytoestrogens. Serve with brown rice.

SERVES 4

$1/3$ cup light soy sauce
$1/3$ cup fresh unsweetened orange juice
1 tablespoon rice vinegar
1 tablespoon sesame oil
1 garlic clove, finely chopped
2 tablespoons chopped cilantro
2 tablespoons finely chopped ginger
$1/2$ teaspoon finely chopped chile
1 head bok choy
1 pound firm tofu, drained and cut in 1-inch cubes
   (about 4 cups)
20 shiitake or button mushrooms
1 red onion, cut lengthwise into 8 wedges
Wooden skewers, soaked in water for about 30 minutes

1 Prepare the marinade by combining the first eight ingredients.

2 Separate the bok choy leaves and cut the stems into 1-inch sections. Marinate with the tofu, mushrooms, and onion for up to 1 hour, depending upon how strong a flavor you want.

3 Thread the ingredients (you'll need to roll the bok choy leaves) onto four large (or twelve small) thick wooden skewers, and cook on a barbecue or under a broiler for 7–10 minutes, basting with the marinade and turning regularly.

Per portion: 242 cal., 8g fat, 1.0g sat. fat, 0.02g sodium, 28g carbohydrate

zucchini, sun-dried tomato, and basil frittata

This is a fantastic egg-based dish that is full of Mediterranean flavor and goodness. Serve in wedges, warm or at room temperature.

SERVES 4

1 tablespoon extra-virgin olive oil
1 onion, finely sliced
1 teaspoon fresh thyme leaves
1 large zucchini, cut in half lengthwise and finely sliced
2 ounces sun-dried tomatoes, chopped (about $1/3$ cup if
   packed in oil or $1/2$ cup if from dried package)
1 cup canned borlotti or kidney beans (canned in
   water), drained and rinsed
3 tablespoons torn basil leaves
6 eggs, lightly beaten
Ground black pepper

1 Heat half the oil in a 9-inch nonstick frying pan and cook the onion and thyme over medium heat until the onion has softened but is still colorless. Add the zucchini and cook for another 3–5 minutes until tender.

2 Pour the mixture into a colander to drain and cool, then combine with the sun-dried tomatoes, beans, and basil. Add this mixture to the beaten egg, and season with ground black pepper.

3 Wipe the frying pan with paper towels, then pour in the remaining oil and place over medium heat. When the oil is hot enough to make the egg sizzle, pour in the egg mixture. Stir with a fork for a couple of minutes to ensure that the pan is evenly covered. Reduce the heat and cook the frittata gently until the bottom is lightly set, about 10 minutes.

4 Slide the frittata onto a large plate, then lay the frying pan, upside-down, over the plate, hold together tightly, and turn the whole thing upside-down so the frittata is inverted in the pan. Cook for another 5 minutes until just firm.

Per portion: 269 cal., 19g fat, 3.9g sat. fat, 0.36g sodium, 11g carbohydrate

chickpea curry

Try making this curry instead of a dal. Like all savory stews, it is best eaten the day after making, so that the flavors have time to mellow.

SERVES 6–8

*1²/3 cups dried chickpeas, soaked overnight then drained
  and rinsed
1-inch piece of ginger, peeled and sliced
3 bay leaves
3-inch piece of cinnamon stick
3 large onions, roughly chopped
2 tablespoons olive oil
1 tablespoon finely chopped garlic
1 tablespoon grated ginger
1 teaspoon ground turmeric
2 chiles, seeded and finely sliced
One x 14¹/2-ounce can of chopped tomatoes
2 crushed black or green cardamoms
6 whole cloves
1 teaspoon black peppercorns
1 teaspoon cumin seeds, toasted
1 cauliflower, broken into florets
8-ounce bag washed spinach (about 4 large handfuls)
1 tablespoon garam masala
1 tablespoon chopped fresh mint
2 tablespoons chopped cilantro*

1 Cook the chickpeas with the sliced ginger, bay leaves, two thirds of the cinnamon stick, and half the onion in about 8 cups water until tender. This will take about 1–2 hours, depending upon the age of the chickpeas. Drain, reserving the liquid, and discard the ginger, bay leaves, and cinnamon.

2 Meanwhile, 45 minutes before the chickpeas have finished cooking, blend the remaining onions in a food processor. Heat the olive oil in a large pot, then cook the onions with the garlic and ginger until the onions have softened but not yet colored.

3 Add the turmeric and chiles and cook for another 3 minutes. Add the canned tomatoes and half of the reserved cooking liquid and bring to a boil.

4 Tie the remaining cinnamon, cardamom, cloves, peppercorns, and cumin in cheesecloth and add to the tomatoes. Bring to a simmer, then add the cauliflower and cook for about 20 minutes.

5 Add the spinach, stir to combine, and cook until the spinach has wilted. Add the drained chickpeas and simmer for another 15 minutes. Add as much of the remaining chickpea cooking liquid as needed to give the preferred consistency. Remove and squeeze the juices from the cheesecloth. Stir in the garam masala, mint and cilantro.

6 Serve with brown basmati rice or whole-wheat chapatis.

Per portion: 186 cal., 7g fat, 0.9g sat. fat, 0.09g sodium, 23g carbohydrate

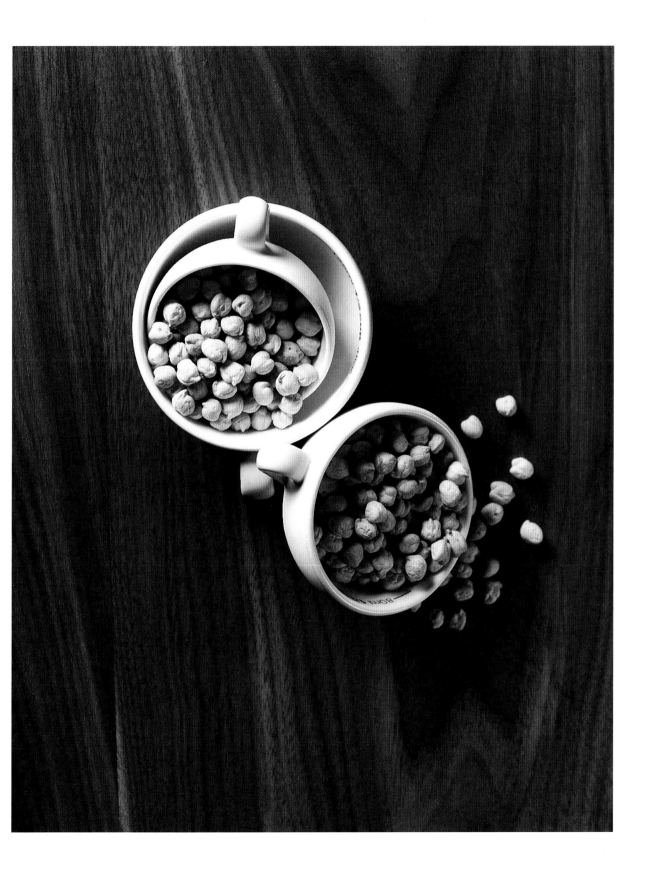

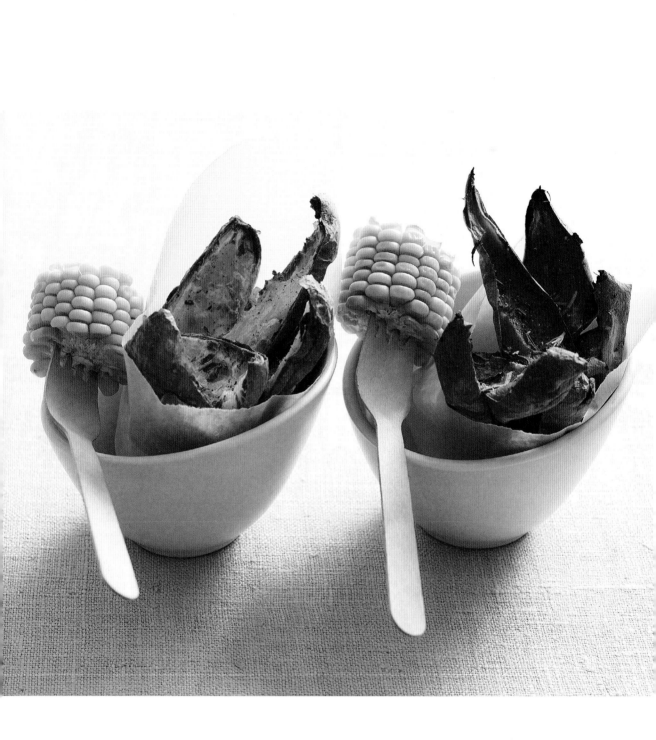

baked potato skins

Simply irresistible, these will make your mouth water as they cook. Eat with corn or refried beans for a nutritious, low-G.I. snack.

SERVES 4

6 potatoes or sweet potatoes, each about 6 ounces
1 tablespoon olive oil
Salt and ground black pepper
1 tablespoon finely chopped fresh rosemary

1 Preheat the oven to 400°F.

2 Prick each potato all over and place them directly on the oven shelf. Bake for 40–45 minutes or until slightly softened when squeezed, then let cool.

3 Cut each potato in half lengthwise and then in half again. Slice away a bit of the flesh, leaving a layer of potato at least 1/4-inch thick on the skin. Brush the skins with oil, then arrange in a single layer, skin side down, on a wire rack set in a roasting pan. Season with salt and pepper, and sprinkle the rosemary over it. Bake for about 30 minutes until crisp and golden brown. Serve hot.

Per portion: 222 cal., 3g fat, 0.4g sat. fat, 0.22g sodium, 45g carbohydrate

corn and pepper bake

This is a really satisfying dish based on a traditional southern American recipe. Serve with whole-grain bread or grilled chicken.

SERVES 6

1 tablespoon olive oil
2 leeks, shredded
1 red pepper, seeded and chopped
14 ounces frozen corn (about 1^2/$_3$ cups), thawed and well drained
Ground black pepper
4 eggs
1 teaspoon English mustard
2^1/$_2$ cups 2% or low-fat milk
^{1}/$_2$ teaspoon Tabasco sauce
^{1}/$_2$ teaspoon Worcestershire sauce

1 Preheat the oven to 350°F.

2 Heat the oil in a large saucepan and cook the leeks, red pepper, and corn for 5 minutes. Season generously with black pepper and pour the mixture into a baking dish.

3 In a bowl, beat together the eggs, mustard, milk, and Tabasco and Worcestershire sauces. Pour this over the corn mixture. Bake in a hot water bath for 35–40 minutes or until a knife comes out clean when inserted into the center.

Per portion: 148 cal., 8g fat, 2.5g sat. fat, 0.79g sodium, 9g carbohydrate

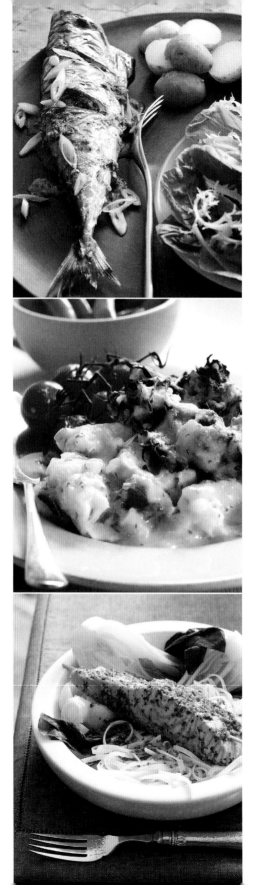

fish

seared swordfish with salsa fresca

Swordfish are found in temperate as well as tropical waters and are extremely popular in the US. Best grilled, this meaty fish isn't overpowered by the spicy salsa. Serve with new potatoes in their skins and a green salad.

SERVES 4

1 teaspoon olive oil
1 garlic clove, finely chopped
1 red chile, seeded and finely chopped
1/2 teaspoon ground cumin
1/2 teaspoon ground coriander
Juice of 1 lime
Ground black pepper
41/2 ounce swordfish steaks
5 ounces tiny cherry tomatoes, cut in half (about 1 cup)
1 ripe, firm avocado, peeled, pitted and chopped
1 very small red onion, finely chopped
2 tablespoons chopped fresh cilantro

1 Place the oil in a shallow non-metallic dish with the garlic, half the chile, half the ground cumin, and half the ground coriander. Add half the lime juice, and season with pepper. Stir well, then add the swordfish steaks, turning to coat. Cover with plastic wrap and marinate for 30 minutes to let the flavors develop.

2 To make the salsa, place the remaining chile, ground cumin, coriander, and lime juice in a bowl. Add the cherry tomatoes, avocado, red onion, and fresh cilantro and mix gently to combine. Set aside.

3 Heat a grill pan. Remove the swordfish steaks from the marinade. Add to the pan and charbroil for 1–2 minutes on each side or until well seared and just tender.

4 Spoon some salsa over the swordfish and serve at once.

Per portion: 226 cal., 13g fat, 2.8g sat. fat, 0.17g sodium, 3g carbohydrate

seared tuna sashimi with spicy lentil salad

In Japan, sashimi is a dish of sliced raw fish that is traditionally presented on a pile of shredded radish with wasabi and a dipping sauce. Here, the tuna is lightly seared and served on a bed of lentils. Lentils contain considerably more protein than any other vegetable as well as being full of fiber. Adding them to a dish will lower the G.I. Pregnant women, nursing mothers, and the elderly are not advised to eat raw fish.

SERVES 4–6

4 teaspoons black peppercorns, quite finely ground and mixed with 1/4 teaspoon powdered star anise
1 pound very fresh trimmed tuna loin (preferably sashimi grade, otherwise buy from a good fish market), in one piece
2–4 teaspoons wasabi paste (Japanese green horseradish)
6 tablespoons reduced-calorie mayonnaise

Spicy lentil salad
9 ounces (about 11/4 cups) French lentils, washed
Vegetable broth or water
3 garlic cloves
11/2 red onions, finely chopped
Finely grated zest and juice of 1 lime
1 tablespoon extra-virgin olive oil
4 large red chiles, charbroiled or roasted, seeded and chopped
Cilantro leaves, for garnishing

Dipping sauce
5 tablespoons light soy sauce
1/2 teaspoon juices from grated fresh ginger
1/2 teaspoon wasabi paste

1 Place the black pepper mix in a shallow tray and roll the tuna in it, pressing the pepper into the flesh. Heat a thick bottomed frying pan without fat over a high heat until extremely hot. Place the tuna in the pan and sear each side until the heat has penetrated 1/4-inch all around. The pepper will be nicely charred and aromatic. Set aside and, when cool, refrigerate until ready to serve.

2 Mix the wasabi paste into the mayonnaise until the desired fieriness is achieved.

3 To make the lentil salad, put the lentils in a saucepan and add the broth or water until it covers the lentils by about one inch. Cook with the whole garlic over medium heat for 20–25 minutes until just tender. Drain, discard the garlic, and fold in the remaining ingredients.

4 To make the dipping sauce, mix the ingredients together with 5 tablespoons iced water and leave for 30 minutes.

5 Remove the tuna from the fridge and cut it into $3/8$-inch slices using a simple, single draw from top to bottom with a long, sharp knife. The flesh of the tuna will cut like butter so do not be tempted to use a sawing motion.

6 To serve, place a heap of lentils on each plate. Lean the slices of tuna against the lentils. Garnish with cilantro leaves and serve with the dipping sauce and wasabi mayonnaise.

Per portion: 494 cal., 18g fat, 3.2g sat. fat, 0.52g sodium, 41g carbohydrate

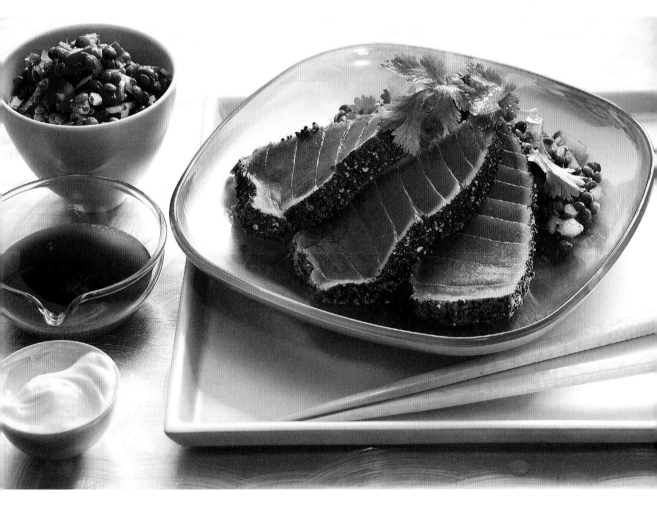

300+

grilled tuna with celeriac skordalia and arugula

Skordalia is a Greek garlic sauce, usually made with bread or potatoes. The key to making it successfully is to add the olive oil slowly. I've added celeriac as well, as it is a lovely mild, slightly sweet-tasting vegetable that is full of fiber and goes really well with potatoes.

SERVES 4

Celeriac skordalia
12 ounces peeled celeriac (celery root), cubed (about 3 cups)
4 ounces new potatoes, unpeeled and cubed, (about 3/4 cups)
5 garlic cloves, finely chopped
1 tablespoon lemon juice or white wine vinegar
2 tablespoons extra-virgin olive oil
Ground black pepper

4 tuna loin steaks, about 41/2 ounces each
1 tablespoon extra-virgin olive oil
Ground black pepper
4 handfuls arugula leaves, washed and dried
4 lemon wedges

1 For the skordalia, steam the celeriac and potatoes for about 20 minutes until tender. Soak the garlic in the lemon juice.

2 Put the warm vegetables in a food processor and blend until smooth. With the machine running, add the garlic and slowly pour in the oil as if you were making a mayonnaise. Season to taste with the pepper and the lemon juice.

3 To cook the tuna, preheat a ridged grill pan. Rub the tuna lightly with olive oil and pepper. Cook for 1–2 minutes on each side, depending upon how rare you like the tuna. (It's up to you, but I think well-done tuna is a waste and you may as well just open a can.)

4 Serve the tuna on the celeriac skordalia with the arugula on the side and a wedge of lemon.

Per portion: 300 cal., 15g fat, 2.9g sat. fat, 0.14g sodium, 9g carbohydrate

pan-fried mullet with olives and tomatoes

Quick and easy, this is a perfect supper recipe. Although this dish is based on Mediterranean cooking, red mullet is also found in the Atlantic. Serve with new potatoes in their skins and green beans.

SERVES 2

2 tablespoons black olive puree
2 medium-sized red mullet (or red snapper), filleted
1 tablespoon extra-virgin olive oil
9 ounces tomatoes, seeded and chopped
4 teaspoons coarsely chopped tarragon or chervil (about 1 cup)
1 tablespoon chopped basil
Ground black pepper
Juice of 1/2–1 lime

1 Spread the olive puree on the flesh side of the fish.

2 Heat the olive oil in a nonstick frying pan and cook the fillets, skin side up, for 3 minutes. Turn the fillets over and cook for another 3 minutes. Remove and keep warm.

3 Combine the tomatoes, herbs, and pepper, and warm through in the frying pan, adding lime juice to taste. Pour this dressing over the red mullet, and serve.

Per portion: 186 cal., 10g fat, 1.0g sat. fat, 0.22g sodium, 4g carbohydrate

112 | The Recipes

spaghetti with anchovies and parsley

This dish is packed with taste but is really easy to make. Perfect for when you want a quick meal, this is also a great standby to make with ingredients already in store.

SERVES 4

12 ounces dried spaghetti
6 garlic cloves, smashed roughly with the back of a knife
2-ounce can anchovies, chopped—reserve the oil
2 chiles, seeded and finely sliced
6 tablespoons chopped parsley
2 tablespoons dry white wine
¹/₂–1 teaspoon ground black pepper

1 Cook the spaghetti in plenty of boiling water until cooked but still *al dente*. When the pasta is cooked, drain and return to the pot, reserving a little pasta water.

2 Meanwhile, fry the garlic, anchovies, and chiles in the reserved anchovy oil from the can in a medium frying pan over gentle heat for about 10 minutes until the garlic is golden.

3 Add the parsley, white wine, pepper, and a ¹/₄ cup pasta water to deglaze the pan (ie., heat the mixture and stir to loosen any bits stuck to the pan).

4 Pour the anchovy mixture over the pasta and toss to combine, adding a little extra reserved water if necessary.

Per portion: 347 cal., 4g fat, 0.0g sat. fat, 0.50g sodium, 66g carbohydrate

herbed trout with fennel

Trout is an excellent source of omega-3 fatty acids, and is also full of flavor. It needs nothing more than a few salad greens and lemon to accompany it.

SERVES 2

4 sprigs of rosemary
4 sprigs of fennel fronds
4 sprigs of parsley
4 sprigs of oregano
2 medium-sized trout, gutted
1 tablespoon olive oil
Ground black pepper
2 small heads fennel, cut in 2 lengthwise
Handful of arugula leaves
Lemon wedges

1 Preheat the oven to 375°F.

2 Place the herbs inside the trout and tie with fine string or secure with wooden toothpicks.

3 Arrange the fish in a shallow flameproof roasting pan. Drizzle the olive oil over the fish and season with pepper.

4 Blanch the fennel in boiling water for 10 minutes, then drain and place next to the trout. Brown the trout and fennel over medium heat on top of the stove, turning once, then transfer to the oven for about 15 minutes to finish cooking.

5 Serve the trout with the fennel and pour any cooking juices over it, along with some arugula leaves and lemon wedges.

Per portion: 363 cal., 18g fat, 3.3g sat. fat, 0.12g sodium, 4g carbohydrate

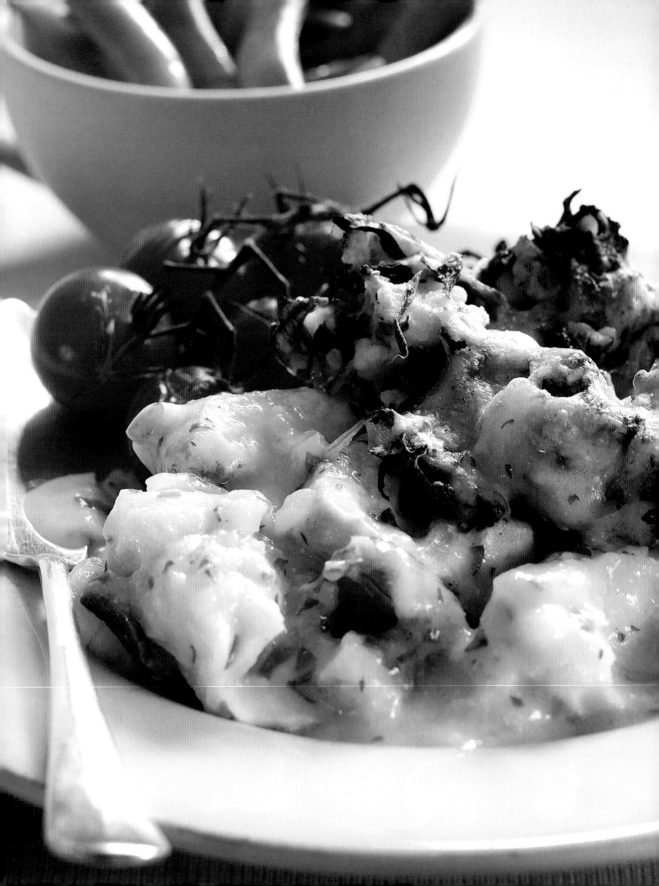

smoked haddock, salmon, and shrimp pie with a spinach topping

A fish pie is one of the most comforting meals and this version is no exception. Full of aromatic herbs and spices with a golden cheesy top, I make this when I need a really filling meal. The mashed potato has been combined with spinach to bring down the G.I., and to add a good source of iron and fiber and give it a lovely speckly appearance.

SERVES 6

18 ounces starchy potatoes, cut into chunks (about 3 1/2–4 cups)
18 ounces frozen spinach, thawed and thoroughly drained (about 2–2 1/2 cups)
3 cups skim milk
Grated fresh nutmeg
Ground black pepper
2 fresh bay leaves
1 whole clove
9-ounce salmon fillet (in one piece)
9-ounce haddock fillet (in one piece)
2 tablespoons unsalted butter
1 onion, finely chopped
1/4 cup cornstarch
1 teaspoon anchovy paste
2 tablespoons chopped fresh parsley
1/2 teaspoon fresh thyme leaves
1 teaspoon dry English mustard powder
7 ounces large peeled shrimp (raw or cooked)—about 2 cups
2 ounces Gruyère (or Swiss) cheese, grated (about 1/2 cup)
1 ounce freshly grated Parmesan (about 1/2 cup)
Sugar snap peas (if unavailable, use snow peas or frozen peas)
Roasted cherry tomatoes

1 Preheat the oven to 400°F.

2 To make the topping, steam the potatoes for 15–20 minutes or until completely tender. Drain and return to the pan along with the thawed spinach and heat over low for a couple of minutes to dry out, shaking the pan occasionally to prevent the potatoes sticking to the bottom. Mash the potatoes, then beat in up to 1/2 cup milk and season to taste with nutmeg and pepper.

3 Place 2 1/2 cups milk in a sauté pan or frying pan, along with the bay leaves, clove, and a pinch of nutmeg. Add the salmon and haddock fillets and poach for 6–8 minutes or until the fish is just tender. Transfer the fish fillets to a plate and set aside until they are cool enough to handle, then flake the flesh, discarding the skin and any bones. Set aside. Strain the poaching liquid and set aside.

4 Melt the butter in a large nonstick pan. Add the onion and cook for 6–8 minutes until the onion has softened but not colored, stirring occasionally. Pour in the reserved poaching milk. Mix the cornstarch to a paste with 1/2 cup water, then add a little warm milk from the pan and return to the rest of the liquid, stirring all the time. Reduce the heat and simmer gently for 10 minutes, stirring occasionally until slightly reduced and thickened.

5 Stir the anchovy paste, parsley, thyme, and mustard powder into the sauce. Fold in the reserved flaked fish and shrimp, then season to taste. Spoon the fish mixture into an ovenproof dish, that is at least 2 1/2 quarts in size. Let a light skin form, then carefully spread the spinach and potato mash over it to cover. Smooth the top with a spatula and fluff up with a fork. Mix together the Gruyère and Parmesan and sprinkle them over the top, then bake for 20–25 minutes or until the cheese is bubbling and golden.

6 Serve at once with the vegetables.

Per portion: 370 cal., 14g fat, 5.9g sat. fat, 0.41g sodium, 28g carbohydrate

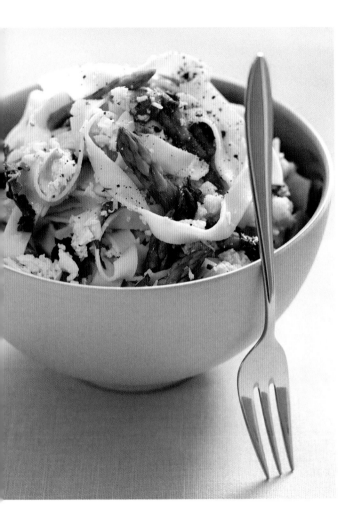

crab and asparagus fettuccine

Pasta is one of the best G.I. foods. Low in fat, it will also fill you up and prevent late-night snacking. White crab meat comes from the claws, but you can also use brown meat—it has a more intense flavor.

SERVES 4

2 tablespoons extra-virgin olive oil
1 shallot, finely chopped (if unavailable, use
    1 tablespoon minced mild onion)
1 tablespoon lemon thyme leaves
2 teaspoons anchovy paste
$^2/_3$ cup dry white wine
$^2/_3$ cup fish stock
12 ounces asparagus, trimmed and cut into 1-inch pieces
    (about 3–3$^1/_2$ cups)
9 ounces white crabmeat (about 1$^1/_4$–1$^1/_2$ cups)
14 ounces fresh fettuccine (about 2$^1/_2$–3 cups)
2 teaspoons unsalted butter
Juice of 1 lemon
$^1/_4$ cup chopped fresh parsley
Ground black pepper

1 Heat the olive oil in a heavy frying pan, add the shallot, and cook gently until soft but not brown. Add the thyme, anchovy paste, wine, and fish stock, and bring to a boil. Reduce to a simmer.

2 Meanwhile bring a large pot of water to a boil. Add the asparagus and cook for 4–6 minutes until just tender. Drain, reserving the cooking water, and add the asparagus to the shallot liquid along with the crab.

3 Cook the fettuccine in the asparagus water for 3–4 minutes. Drain and add to the crab sauce.

4 Heat the butter in a frying pan until nutty and golden. Add the lemon juice and parsley and pour it over the pasta. Toss to combine. Season to taste with plenty of black pepper.

Per portion: 476 cal., 16g fat, 3.3g sat. fat, 0.74g sodium, 50g carbohydrate

thai steamed salmon

Here the salmon is marinated in cilantro, ginger, mint, lime juice, and chiles. Serve with brown basmati rice or rice noodles and steamed green beans or bok choy.

SERVES 4

Small bunch of cilantro, washed
12 mint leaves, washed
1/2 teaspoon salt
2 garlic cloves, crushed
2 green chiles, seeded and chopped
3 tablespoons fresh lime juice
1 tablespoon sugar
1 teaspoon peeled and chopped fresh ginger
1 tablespoon fish sauce (Nam Pla)
4 1/2 ounce salmon fillets

1 In a food processor, blend together the cilantro leaves and stalks, mint leaves, salt, garlic, and chiles to make a rough paste. Add the lime juice, sugar, ginger, and fish sauce, and blend until fairly smooth. Spoon the sauce into a heatproof bowl and combine with the salmon, then marinate for 20 minutes.

2 Boil some water in the bottom half of a steamer. Place the bowl with the marinated salmon in the top half and steam for 6–8 minutes.

3 Serve immediately with the rice or noodles and vegetables.

Per portion: 254 cal., 14g fat, 2.4g sat. fat, 0.37g sodium, 7g carbohydrate

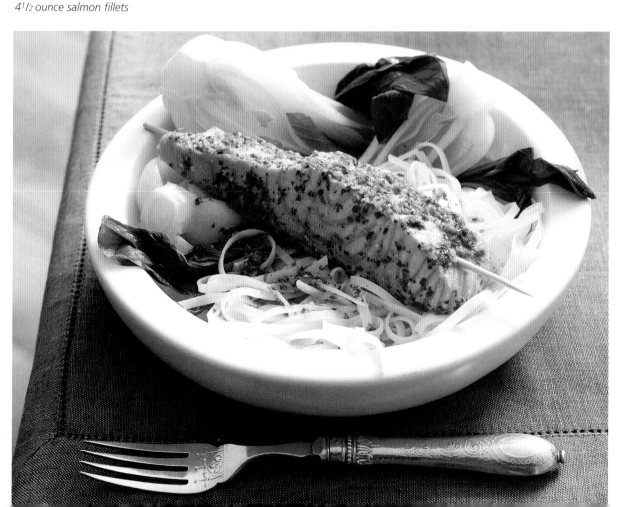

thai fish cakes with cucumber relish

SERVES 4

Cucumber relish
1/2 cup rice vinegar (if unavailable, use apple cider vinegar)
2 tablespoons sugar
4-inch piece cucumber, unpeeled
1 small carrot
1 shallot, finely sliced
1 red chile, seeded and finely sliced
2 tablespoons roasted peanuts, roughly chopped

18 ounces cod fillet, skinned
1 ounce fresh cilantro, chopped (about 2 cups)
2–3 tablespoons red curry paste
1 teaspoon cornstarch mixed with 1 tablespoon lime juice
1 egg white
2 scallions, finely chopped
Oil spray, for frying

1 To make the relish, boil the vinegar and sugar until the sugar dissolves, simmer for 1–2 minutes, then let cool.

2 Quarter the cucumber lengthwise, seed then slice crosswise finely. Cut the carrot in half lengthwise and slice thinly.

3 Add the cucumber, carrot, shallot, and chile to the cold syrup and mix. Leave for 4 hours. Add the peanuts before serving.

4 Put all the ingredients for the fish cakes except the scallions and oil in a food processor and blend until the mixture forms a somewhat smooth paste. Remove from the food processor and work in the scallions.

5 Spray a nonstick frying pan with oil and cook a small amount of the mixture to check the seasoning. If you like, add more curry paste, then shape the mixture into 12 small cakes. Fry the fish cakes for about 3 minutes each side until cooked through. Serve warm with the relish.

Per portion: 239 cal., 8g fat, 1.1g sat. fat, 0.25g sodium, 15g carbohydrate

mussels with bacon

This is full of wonderful tastes and aromas. Serve with whole-grain bread or brown basmati rice to soak up all the cooking liquor, and a green salad.

SERVES 4

2/3 cup hard (alcoholic) cider (if unavailable, use dry white wine)
4 1/2 pounds fresh mussels, cleaned and beards removed
4 slices Canadian bacon (back bacon), cut in thin strips
1/2 onion, finely chopped
6 sage leaves, finely chopped
1 red apple, cored and chopped
Ground black pepper

1 In a very large pot, bring the cider to a fast boil, add the mussels, and cover with a lid. Cook for 3–5 minutes, shaking the pot occasionally, until the mussels open. Discard any that remain closed. Remove about half the mussels from their shells if you wish, and reserve the cooking liquid.

2 Strain the mussel liquor, return it to the heat, add the mussels, and keep on the gentlest simmer.

3 Meanwhile, in a frying pan, cook the bacon with the onion and sage until the bacon is crisp. Add the apple and cook for another 2–3 minutes. Season with ground black pepper.

4 Divide the mussels with their liquor between four warm bowls. Sprinkle the bacon mixture over them and eat with warm whole-grain bread or brown basmati rice.

Per portion: 252 cal., 7g fat, 1.8g sat. fat, 1.13g sodium, 10g carbohydrate

moroccan mussels with spices

SERVES 4

1 tablespoon olive oil
1 small onion, chopped
2 garlic cloves, chopped
2 tablespoons chopped fresh cilantro
1/2 teaspoon dried chiles, crushed
1 teaspoon paprika
1 teaspoon ground cumin
2 tomatoes, chopped
1 tablespoon tomato paste
2/3 cup tomato juice
2 1/3 pounds mussels, cleaned and beards removed
1/2 teaspoon grated lemon zest
2–3 teaspoons lemon juice
2 tablespoons chopped fresh flat-leaf parsley
6 lemon wedges
Ground black pepper

1 Heat a large saucepan over a high heat, add the olive oil, onion, and garlic, and stir.

2 Add the cilantro, chiles, paprika, cumin, 2/3 cup water, tomatoes, tomato paste, and tomato juice, and stir continuously. Bring to a boil.

3 Add the cleaned mussels and stir well, ensuring that all the mussels are well coated in sauce. Cover and simmer for 5–8 minutes, shaking occasionally (or until the mussels have opened). Add the lemon zest and juice to taste, and season with pepper if wished.

4 Garnish with parsley and lemon wedges, and serve at once with baked potato skins or oven-baked fries, and a fresh green salad.

Per portion: 126 cal., 5g fat, 0.7g sat. fat, 0.35g sodium, 8g carbohydrate

smoked monkfish

Monkfish is a firm white fish, ideal for this dish as it keeps its shape and absorbs the flavors of the spices well. Shrimp are a good alternative—use raw, peeled shrimp and stir fry for about 3 minutes until completely pink, and no longer translucent.

SERVES 4

1 tablespoon vegetable oil
1 teaspoon five-spice powder
1 red onion, finely chopped
1-inch cube fresh root ginger, peeled and chopped
2–3 large garlic cloves, crushed
1/2 teaspoon chile powder
1/2 teaspoon fennel seeds, toasted in a dry skillet, then ground
2 teaspoons tomato puree
1 pound monkfish, cleaned and cut into 2-inch chunks
    or 450g (1lb) raw shrimp, peeled
1 tablespoon lemon juice
2 tablespoons finely chopped fresh cilantro leaves

1 Heat the oil in a small saucepan over low to medium heat and add the five-spice powder. Let the spices sizzle gently for 35–40 seconds before adding the onion. Fry for 5–6 minutes, then add the ginger and garlic, and cook for a further 1–2 minutes.

2 Add the chile powder, and ground fennel, and cook for 1 minute, then add the tomato puree. Stir once, and add the monkfish or shrimp. Continue to cook for 6–8 minutes, until the fish is cooked through.

3 Stir in the lemon juice and cilantro leaves, and serve with brown basmati rice or heavily seeded flat bread or rolls, and a fresh green salad.

Per portion: 121 cal., 4g fat, 0.4g sat. fat, 0.04g sodium, 5g carbohydrate

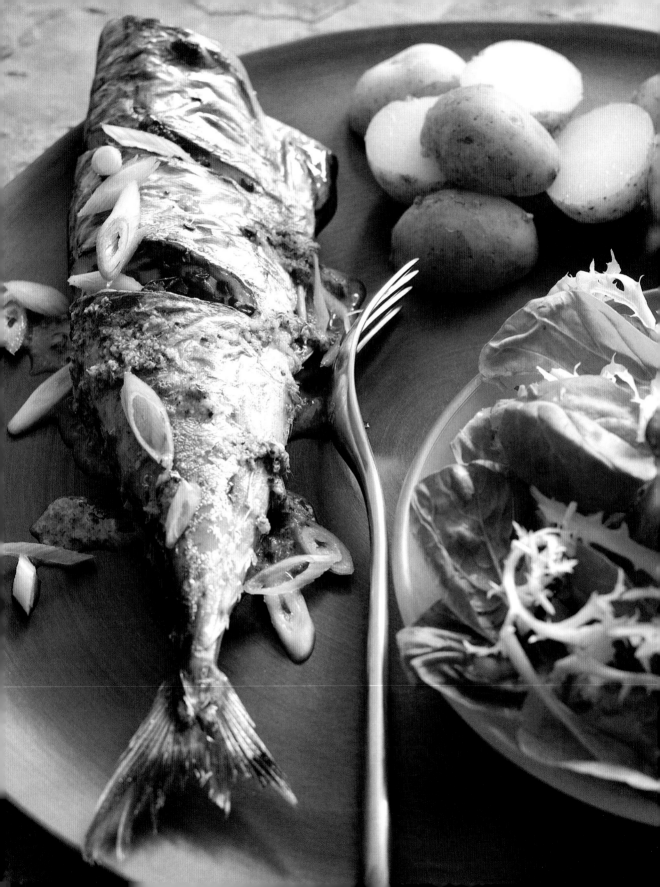

broiled mackerel with chile and horseradish

Fresh mackerel can be quite hard to find, but well worth the effort. It is a beautiful-looking fish with silver-gray markings and a fantastic flavor. It also contains more omega-3 fatty acids than any other fish. Serve with new potatoes in their skins and a green vegetable or salad.

SERVES 4

4 very fresh small whole mackerel, heads removed, gutted, and well cleaned
1 tablespoon seeded and chopped red chile
Ground black pepper
1 tablespoon olive oil
4 scallions, finely sliced
4 teaspoons grated horseradish (not creamed)
1 teaspoon dried red pepper flakes
2 teaspoons chopped fresh rosemary leaves
Juice of 2 lemons

1 Slash the mackerel twice on each side, and place a little chopped chile in each cut. Season with black pepper and rub with the olive oil.

2 Place the fish under a hot broiler or on a barbecue (weather permitting). Cook for 5–7 minutes each side or until the skin is crispy and the fish is cooked through.

3 Meanwhile mix the scallions, horseradish, red pepper flakes, and rosemary, then add the lemon juice and a dash of water to give a pouring consistency.

4 Drizzle this over the mackerel and serve.

Per portion: 249 cal., 19g fat, 3.7g sat. fat, 0.08g sodium, 1g carbohydrate

broiled squid with marinated belgian endive

Scoring the squid before cooking not only makes the finished result look more professional, it also helps the squid to cook through quickly and the shorter the cooking time, the more tender the end result will be.

SERVES 4

1 scant cup (7 fluid ounces) cider vinegar
2^1/$_2$ tablespoons sugar
1 chile, sliced in half
Sprig of thyme
1 bay leaf
1 teaspoon black peppercorns, crushed
1 teaspoon juniper berries, crushed
4 heads Belgian endive
2 tablespoons extra-virgin olive oil
3 tablespoons chopped flat-leaf parsley
Ground black pepper
14 ounces prepared and cleaned squid
2 teaspoons chopped fresh red chile

1 Pour 4 cups water into a nonreactive saucepan, add the vinegar, sugar, and flavorings and bring to a boil. Add the endive to this marinade and cook for 10 minutes.

2 Drain well, then cut the endive in half lengthwise. Drizzle the endive with half the oil and scatter with parsley. Season to taste with black pepper and let cool to room temperature.

3 Lightly slash the squid at 1/2-inch intervals without cutting all the way through.

4 Toss the squid in the remaining oil, then place it on a preheated ridged grill pan and cook for no more than 1 minute each side, depending upon its thickness. Season with pepper and sprinkle with the chopped chile. Serve with the endive.

Per portion: 196 cal., 8g fat, 1.3g sat. fat, 0.13g sodium, 13g carbohydrate

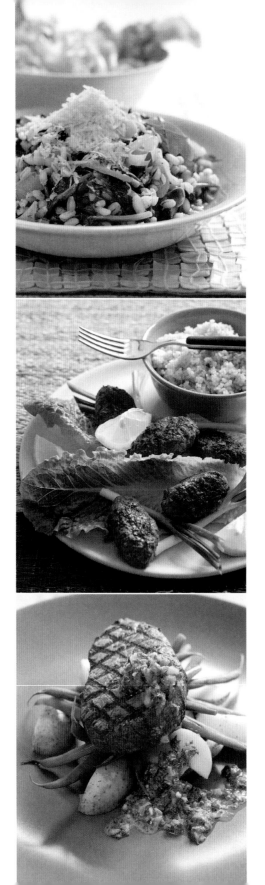

meat and poultry

spicy chicken fillets

You need to marinate the chicken overnight in the spices, but it is worth planning ahead as the marinade keeps the chicken from drying out under the broiler and gives it lots of flavor.

SERVES 4

4 garlic cloves, crushed
²/₃ cup low-fat plain yogurt
1 tablespoon grated onion
1 chile, seeded and finely chopped
1 teaspoon each of ground coriander, cumin, fenugreek,
    paprika, and ginger
Pinch of dry mustard powder
4 chicken breast fillets, cut in large strips
Lime wedges

1 Mix together the garlic, yogurt, onion, chile, spices, and mustard. Add the chicken and marinate overnight.

2 Scrape most of the yogurt from the chicken, and charbroill or broil for 3–4 minutes on each side.

3 Serve with the lime wedges, brown basmati rice, and a green vegetable or salad. Cold, the chicken makes a great filling for sandwiches and tortilla wraps.

Per portion: 163 cal., 2g fat, 0.6g sat. fat, 0.11g sodium, 4g carbohydrate

simple roast chicken

Here is one of the easiest methods of roasting poultry, where the butter makes the skin crisp and golden. Let the chicken rest for 15 minutes before serving to give it time to reabsorb the juices released, so that the meat will be tender and delicious. Serve with baked sweet potatoes and green vegetables. See also page 133 for another great roast recipe.

SERVES 6

1 large free-range chicken (about 3¹/₄ pounds)
2 teaspoons unsalted butter, melted
Several grindings of black pepper
2 sprigs of thyme
1–2 garlic heads, broken into cloves
³/₄ cup dry white wine

1 Preheat the oven to 425°F.

2 Brush the chicken with the butter, then sprinkle with black pepper. Pop the thyme into the cavity of the chicken. Place the chicken in a roasting pan with the garlic cloves and the white wine and roast in the oven for 20 minutes.

3 Reduce the heat to 375°F and roast for another 45 minutes, basting from time to time. Turn off the oven, but leave the chicken in it to rest for 15 minutes before carving and serving with the juices.

Per portion: 127 cal., 3g fat, 1.4g sat. fat, 0.07g sodium, 1g carbohydrate

moroccan lamb stew with pumpkin and pickled lemon

This is one of my favorite recipes, full of color and flavor. Harissa and pickled lemons are an integral part of North African cooking and are a perfect foil for lamb in this satisfying dish. Serve with bulgur or warmed flatbread.

SERVES 4

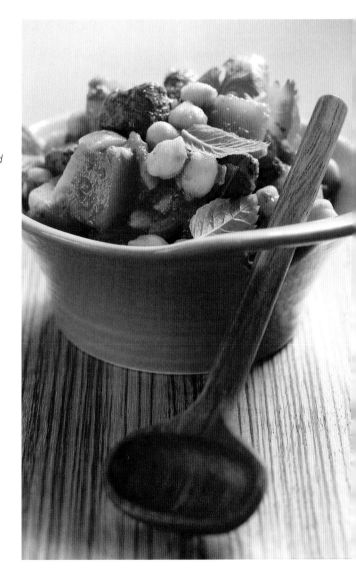

1 pound lean leg of lamb, cut into 1-inch cubes
1 1/2 teaspoons ground black pepper
1 teaspoon olive oil
1 large onion, roughly chopped
4 garlic cloves, crushed
4 tomatoes, skinned and chopped
1 tablespoon harissa or hot pepper paste
One x 15-ounce can of chickpeas in water, drained and rinsed
12 ounces trimmed and peeled pumpkin, cut
    into 1-inch cubes (about 3 cups)
1 pickled lemon, finely chopped
2 tablespoons chopped mint
1 tablespoon chopped cilantro

1 Coat the lamb in the black pepper.

2 Heat the oil in a large nonstick pan, add the lamb, and cook until it has browned all over. Add the onion and garlic and cook until the onion is soft and is slightly brown, adding a splash of water if necessary to prevent sticking.

3 Add the tomatoes, harissa, and 1 3/4 cups water. Bring to a simmer, cover, and cook over medium heat for 1 1/4–1 1/2 hours, topping up with water as necessary, until the lamb is almost tender.

4 Add the chickpeas and pumpkin and cook for another 15 minutes or until the pumpkin is tender. Add the lemon, mint, and cilantro. Serve immediately.

Per portion: 357 cal., 18g fat, 6.6g sat. fat, 0.28g sodium, 21g carbohydrate

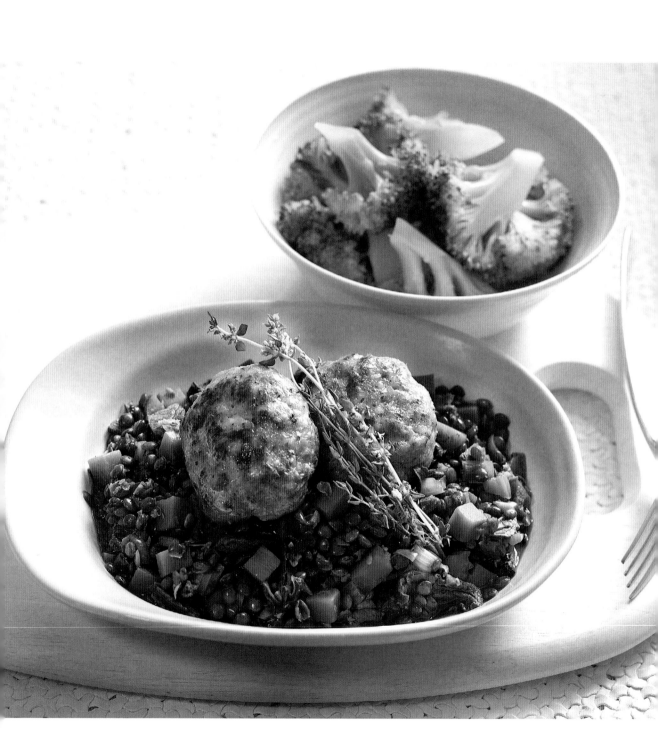

sausage patties with lentils

If you are partial to sausages and mashed potatoes, try this. Instead of mashed potatoes, the lentils make a really flavorsome low-G.I. accompaniment.

SERVES 4

4 ounces smoked Canadian bacon (back bacon), chopped
1 carrot, chopped
1 stalk of celery, chopped
1 onion, chopped
4 garlic cloves, finely chopped
2 teaspoons fresh thyme leaves
1 bay leaf
3 cups chicken broth
2 ounces (50g) dried porcini mushrooms (cèpes) soaked in 1¼ cups boiling water
10 ounces French lentils (about 1⅓ cups), washed
Ground black pepper
1 pound reduced-fat pork sausages (or bulk sausage)

1 Fry the bacon in a nonstick pan until crisp, about 3 minutes. Add the vegetables, garlic, and herbs, and continue to cook until the vegetables have softened, about 5 minutes, adding a dash of water if necessary to prevent sticking.

2 Pour in the chicken broth and bring to a boil. Drain the mushrooms, but reserve the soaking liquid. Squeeze the mushrooms dry and chop roughly, then add to the pan.

3 Pass the mushroom liquid through cheesecloth into the pan. Add the lentils and cook for 20–30 minutes. If the lentils dry out too quickly, add some extra broth. The lentils should be wet but not soupy. Season with black pepper.

4 Meanwhile, shape the bulk sausage into eight patties (or skin the sausages and make patties from the sausage meat). Preheat a broiler and broil cooked through on both sides. Alternatively, just broil the sausages as they are.

5 Serve with the lentils and a green vegetable such as broccoli.

Per portion: 489 cal., 8g fat, 2.6g sat. fat, 0.69g sodium, 64g carbohydrate

pork with ale, black pepper, and prunes

This is wonderful winter food. Marinating the pork and then slow cooking it on the stove and then in the oven infuses this stew with rich, caramelized flavor. Serve with new potatoes in their skins and a green vegetable such as broccoli or cabbage.

SERVES 4

2 teaspoons black peppercorns, crushed
1 teaspoon dried oregano
1 teaspoon fresh thyme leaves
2 garlic cloves, crushed
1 tablespoon raw cane sugar (or regular sugar)
1 tablespoon wine vinegar
4 pork shoulder steaks, each weighing 4½ ounces
2 teaspoons butter
1 onion, finely sliced
1 tablespoon cornstarch
¾ cup strong ale (e.g., Sam Adams)
1 cup chicken broth
12 pitted prunes, cut in half

1 For the marinade, combine the crushed peppercorns, herbs, garlic, sugar, and vinegar.

2 Rub the pork with the marinade, cover, and let marinate in a cool place for at least 3 hours or overnight.

3 Preheat the oven to 350°F.

4 Melt the butter in a heavy flameproof and ovenproof pot and cook the onion over gentle heat until it is lightly golden. Set the pork on top of the onion slices in the pot and lightly brown on both sides. Mix the cornstarch with a little of the ale and add to the pot, then add the rest of the ale and the broth and bring just to a simmer. Add the prunes.

5 Cover, transfer to the oven, and cook for about 1 hour until tender.

Per portion: 274 cal., 8g fat, 3.6g sat. fat, 0.41g sodium, 21g carbohydrate

spaghetti bolognese

There are many ways to make spaghetti bolognese—you can vary the herbs and vegetables, depending upon what you have in stock, or for a vegetarian version, swap the beef and chicken livers for a selection of beans.

SERVES 6

2 ounces Canadian bacon (back bacon), minced (about ¹/3 cup)
1 onion, finely chopped
1 stalk of celery, finely chopped
1 carrot, finely chopped
2 garlic cloves, crushed
1 teaspoon fresh thyme leaves
1 bay leaf
1 teaspoon dried oregano
One x 14¹/2-ounce can of chopped tomatoes
1 tablespoon tomato paste
1 tablespoon Worcestershire sauce
Ground black pepper
12 ounces (about 1¹/2 cups) extra-lean ground beef
   (coarsely ground, if possible)
1 teaspoon olive oil
4 ounces chicken livers (about a heaping ¹/3 cup)
7 fluid ounces (1 scant cup) dry red wine
2¹/2 cups beef broth
18 ounces dried spaghetti
Freshly grated Parmesan, for garnishing (optional)

1 Heat a large, heavy pot and add in the bacon. Cook for a couple of minutes until it is crispy and has released some natural fats, then add the onion, celery, carrot, garlic, thyme, bay leaf, and oregano, and cook over medium heat until the vegetables have softened and taken on a little color, stirring occasionally. Add a dash of water if necessary to prevent sticking.

2 Add the canned tomatoes, tomato paste, and Worcestershire sauce. Stir to combine and season with black pepper to taste.

3 Meanwhile, heat a large nonstick frying pan and fry the ground beef in small batches until browned. While the meat is frying, use a wooden spoon to break up any lumps. Repeat until all the beef is browned. Drain off any fat and stir the meat into the tomato mixture.

4 Wipe out the pan with some paper towels and add the oil, then fry the chicken livers until sizzling and lightly browned. Pour into the ground beef mixture. Then pour some of the red wine into the frying pan, heat it, and scrape any sediment from the bottom. Pour this heated wine and pan scrapings, along with the rest of the wine and the broth into the ground beef mixture, stirring to combine.

5 Bring to a boil, then reduce the heat and simmer, uncovered, stirring from time to time, for about 1 hour until the beef is completely tender and the sauce is rich.

6 To serve, bring a large pot of water to a rolling boil. Swirl in the spaghetti, stir once, and cook for 8–12 minutes or according to package instructions until the pasta is *al dente*. Drain and divide among serving bowls. Pour the sauce over it, scatter some Parmesan on top, if using, and serve immediately.

Per portion: **471 cal., 7g fat, 2.4g sat. fat, 0.66g sodium, 68g carbohydrate**

paprika goulash

A deliciously rich stew with a spicy sweetness from the paprika and caraway. Serve with noodles and a green vegetable such as cabbage, green beans, or broccoli.

SERVES 6

2 tablespoons cornstarch
1 pound, 10 ounces chuck steak, brisket or round, cut into
   1 1/2-inch pieces (about 3–4 cups)
1 tablespoon sunflower oil
2 ounces Canadian bacon (back bacon), chopped (about 1/3 cup)
3 garlic cloves, finely chopped
1 pound onions, grated (about 3–4 cups)
1 tablespoon caraway seeds
1 tablespoon hot smoked paprika, plus extra for garnish
2 1/2 cups beef broth
2 tablespoons tomato paste
Ground black pepper
2/3–1 1/3 cups fat-free yogurt

1 Put the cornstarch and beef into a plastic Ziploc, seal the top, and shake well until all the beef pieces are lightly dusted.

2 Heat the sunflower oil in a heavy pot, add the bacon, garlic, onions, caraway, and paprika, and cook for 3 minutes.

3 Add the beef to the pot, followed by the stock and tomato paste. Season with black pepper. Bring to a simmer, then cover and cook very gently for 2 hours, stirring occasionally, until the meat is tender and the sauce is reduced to a rich consistency.

4 Serve with a generous topping of yogurt sprinkled with paprika.

Per portion: 274 cal., 8g fat, 2.4g sat. fat, 0.38g sodium, 16g carbohydrate

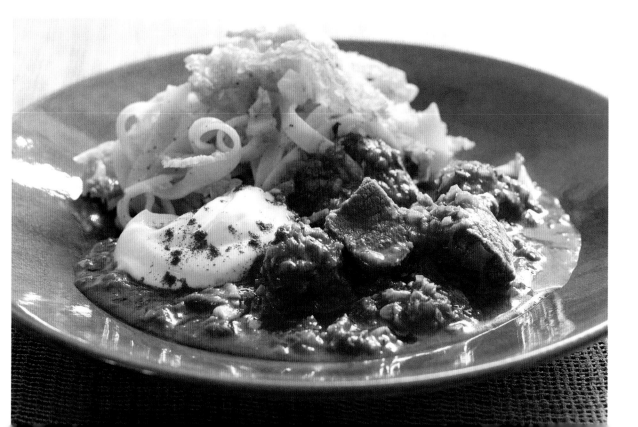

pot-roasted guinea fowl

Game birds contain very little fat, but that means that they dry out easily. This recipe is a great way to avoid that. Serve with green cabbage and new potatoes in their skins or sweet potato.

SERVES 8

2 sprigs of rosemary
2 sprigs of thyme
Two x 2¹/₂ pound guinea fowls or pheasants
Ground black pepper
2 teaspoons unsalted butter
1 tablespoon olive oil
4 slices Canadian bacon (back bacon), chopped
1 large carrot, sliced
1 large onion, chopped
1 stalk of celery, sliced
1 teaspoon fresh thyme leaves
1 cup dry white wine
1³/₄ cups chicken broth

1 Preheat the oven to 425°F.

2 Place the rosemary and thyme in the cavity of the birds. Season the birds with pepper.

3 In a flameproof and ovenproof pot, brown the birds in the butter and olive oil until golden all over. Remove and set aside.

4 To the same pot, add the bacon, carrot, onion, celery, and thyme. Cook until the vegetables have softened and started to brown. Add the wine, scraping any coagulated sediment from the bottom of the pot.

5 Return the birds to the pot, pour in the chicken broth and bring to a simmer. Cover with a lid and place in the oven. Cook for 1–1¹/₂ hours until the thickest part of the thighs is tender when tested with a skewer.

Per portion: 289 cal., 7g fat, 5.1g sat. fat, 0.42g sodium, 4g carbohydrate

tenderloin steak with salsa verde

A good steak is mouthwatering, but we have become more wary of red meat. Try to buy organic, ensure each portion size is no bigger than 4½ ounces, and you can still enjoy it occasionally. Serve with boiled new potatoes in their skins and green beans.

SERVES 4

Small handful flat-leaf parsley
6 basil leaves
¹/₂ small handful mint leaves
1 pickled cucumber
1 garlic clove
1 tablespoon capers, drained and rinsed
2 anchovy fillets, rinsed
¹/₂ tablespoon red wine vinegar
¹/₂ tablespoon fresh lemon juice
¹/₂ tablespoon Dijon mustard
3 tablespoons extra-virgin olive oil
Ground black pepper
Four 4¹/₂-ounce tenderloin steaks

1 Coarsely chop the parsley, basil, mint, and cucumber with the garlic, capers, and anchovy fillets, or pulse in a food processor—but you will get a better result if you chop by hand.

2 Transfer to a non-metallic bowl and whisk in the red wine vinegar, lemon juice, Dijon mustard, all but 1 teaspoon of the olive oil, plus 2 tablespoons cold water. Season with pepper. Set aside, covered with plastic wrap, at room temperature.

3 Heat a heavy frying pan or ridged grill pan. Brush the steaks with the remaining oil and cook for 2–3 minutes on each side, depending upon how rare you like your steak.

4 Transfer the steak to a plate and set aside in a warm place for about 5 minutes. Serve with some salsa verde on the side.

Per portion: 279 cal., 18g fat, 4.7g sat. fat, 0.49g sodium, 1g carbohydrate

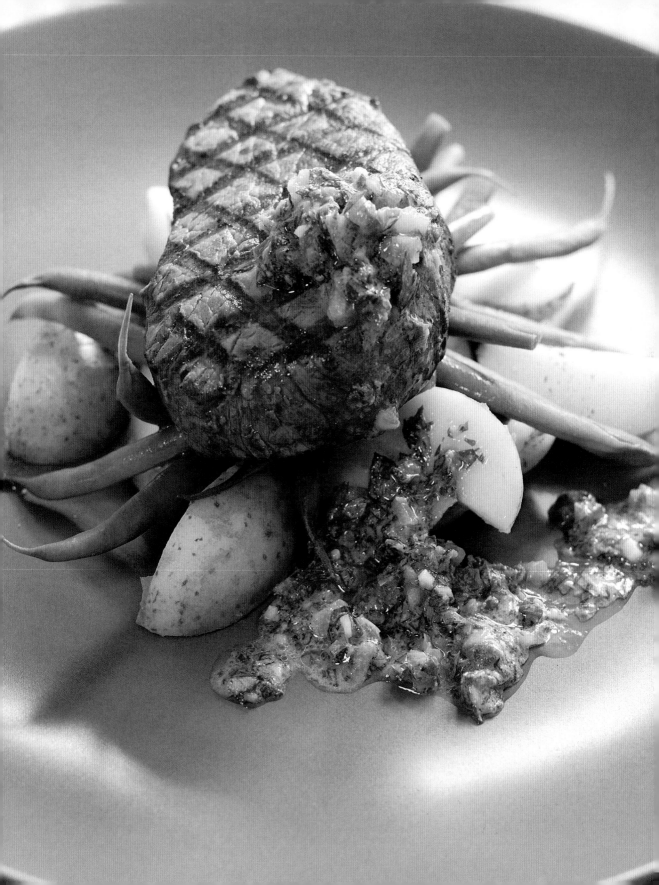

crispy duck with lentils

Although duck contains quite a lot of fat, draining it as it cooks will reduce your intake.

SERVES 6

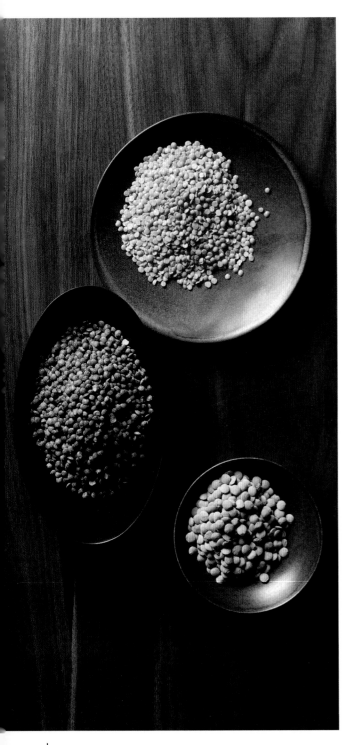

Lentils
12 ounces (about 1³/4 cups) French lentils, washed but
  not soaked
1 onion, finely chopped
1 bay leaf
1 whole clove
1 carrot, chopped
4 ounces Canadian bacon (back bacon), cut in strips
Few sprigs of thyme
2 garlic cloves, peeled
2¹/2 cups chicken broth
1 teaspoon sugar
Ground black pepper

3 large duck breast fillets
1¹/2 teaspoons ground cumin or cinnamon

1 To make the lentils, place them in a pot and cover with cold water. Bring to a boil, drain, and rinse under cold water. Return the lentils to the pot and add the onion, bay leaf, clove, carrot, bacon, thyme, garlic, chicken broth and sugar. Bring to a boil, then reduce the heat, cover the pot, and simmer until the lentils are tender but not mushy, about 20 minutes, adding water as necessary. Drain the lentils if you like but discard the bay leaf, clove, thyme, and garlic. Season with black pepper and keep warm.

2 Meanwhile, cut the skin of the duck in a very close criss-cross pattern and dust with the spice. Place skin side down in a heavy frying pan over medium heat and cook for 10 minutes until the skin is crisp. Pour off any excess fat. Turn the duck skin side up, and cook for another 5–10 minutes to suit your taste. Let rest for 5 minutes, then slice thickly.

3 Pile the lentils onto plates and top with the duck slices.

Per portion: 355 cal., 8g fat, 2.4g sat. fat, 0.54g sodium, 37g carbohydrate

roast turkey

This is a great way to roast a turkey without running the risk of drying the meat, as the herbed butter and cheese pushed under the skin baste the turkey as it cooks. See page 124 for another way to roast poultry.

SERVES 16

4 ounces (about 1/2 cup) ricotta or low-fat cream cheese
1/4 cup (1/2 stick) unsalted butter, softened
1 tablespoon chopped fresh chives
1 tablespoon chopped flat-leaf parsley
1 tablespoon chopped fresh tarragon
1/2 teaspoon sea salt or kosher salt
1/2 teaspoon ground black pepper
One x 10-pound fresh turkey, at room temperature
1 lemon, cut in half
1 onion, cut in half
3 garlic cloves
Sprig of thyme
Sprig of rosemary

1 Preheat the oven to 450°F.

2 Combine the ricotta and butter with the chopped herbs, salt, and pepper.

3 Gently ease the skin covering the turkey breast away from the flesh at both ends by carefully inserting your fingers between the skin and flesh. Push the cheese mixture under the skin, easing it over the whole bird, being careful not to puncture the skin. Place the lemon, onion, garlic, and herb sprigs in the cavity of the turkey.

4 Grease a large sheet of foil and place in a roasting pan lengthwise, leaving enough at each end to wrap over the turkey. Repeat this exercise with another sheet, this time across the roasting pan.

5 Place the turkey, breast-side up in the center of the foil. Wrap the turkey completely in foil and roast for 2 hours. Fold back the foil, making sure the ends of the drumsticks are still covered. Baste the turkey with the juices that have formed in the pan, then cook for another 30 minutes until the turkey is golden brown. Check with a metal skewer to see if the turkey is cooked—the juices in the thickest part of the thigh should run clear.

6 Remove from the oven and let rest in a warm place for 15 minutes to allow the juices to settle and to ease carving. Carefully skim off the fat from the roasting pan and use the remaining meat juices to make gravy, if you like.

Per portion: 295 cal., 13g fat, 5.1g sat. fat, 0.21g sodium, 1g carbohydrate

kofta meatballs

This is a fragrant **Middle Eastern dish where ground meat is flavored with spices and formed into balls. They also freeze well and make a great snack for kids.**

SERVES 4

18 ounces extra-lean beef or lamb, finely ground (about
  2^1/4 cups)
1 onion, finely chopped
2 teaspoons ground cumin
1 teaspoon apple pie spice
Pinch of cayenne pepper
Handful of chopped cilantro leaves
Ground black pepper
1 tablespoon olive oil
Lemon wedges, for serving

1 Blend all the ingredients except the oil and lemon wedges in a food processor until smooth.

2 Take a small handful of the mixture and, using your hands, roll it into a ball or oval shape. Repeat until you have used all the mixture to make 16 meatballs. If you wet your hands first, it will help prevent the mixture from sticking to them.

3 Heat the oil in a large nonstick frying pan and fry the meatballs until they are golden brown and cooked through. Drain on absorbent paper towels and serve with lemon wedges. They are delicious with a green salad and couscous or brown rice.

Per portion: 212 cal., 9g fat, 3.2g sat. fat, 0.08g sodium, 4g carbohydrate

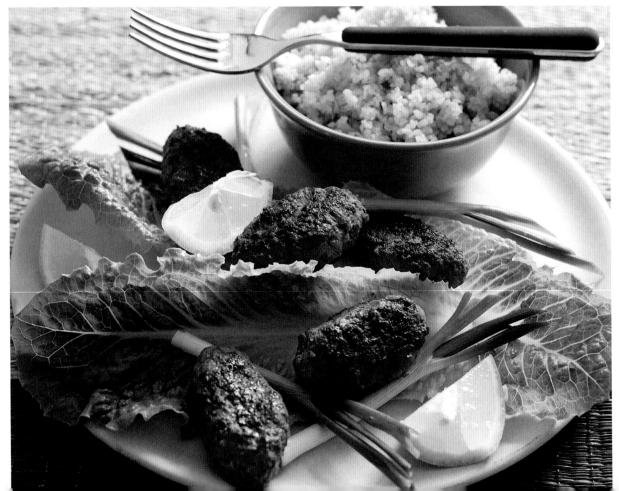

black pudding (blood sausage) with apples

Black pudding, also known as blood sausage, is one of the oldest kinds of sausage in Europe. Love or hate it, it is a good source of iron.

SERVES 4

Crushed white beans
9 ounces (about 1 1/4 cups) dried white beans
1 onion, roughly chopped
1 carrot, chopped
1 stalk of celery, chopped
2 teaspoons chopped garlic
2 ounces ham, roughly chopped (about 1/2 cup)
1 clove
Sprig of thyme
1 bay leaf
1/2 tablespoon ground cumin
1/2 teaspoon ground chili powder

9 ounces (or 8–12 slices) black pudding (preferably a soft
  variety), cut into 1/2-inch slices
1 tablespoon walnut oil
2 shallots, finely chopped (if unavailable, use
  2 tablespoons minced mild onion)
2 dessert apples, e.g., Jonagold or Cortland,
  cored and cut into thin slices
1/4 cup chopped parsley
1 tablespoon cider vinegar
Ground black pepper

1 To prepare the white beans, soak them overnight in plenty of cold water.

2 Rinse the beans, then place in a large pot along with the onion, carrot, celery, garlic, ham, clove, thyme, and bay leaf.

3 Cover with cold water, bring to a boil and simmer until the beans are soft (about 1 hour), adding more water if necessary to keep the beans covered. Drain the beans and remove the clove, thyme, and bay leaf.

4 Crush the beans with a potato masher, then mix in the ground cumin and chili powder.

5 Preheat the broiler to medium and cook the black pudding slices for 2 minutes each side. The slices should be slightly crusty. Remove and set aside, discarding any tough skin.

6 Heat the oil in a medium frying pan and cook the shallots over medium heat until soft but not brown. Add the apple, cook for another 2 minutes, then add the parsley.

7 Pour in the cider vinegar and combine with the other ingredients. Season to taste with pepper.

8 Warm up the bean puree and spoon it onto warmed plates. Top with slices of black pudding and garnish with the apple mixture. Serve immediately.

Per portion: 343 cal., 18g fat, 5.8g sat. fat, 0.74g sodium, 33g carbohydrate

shepherd's pie with a g.i. twist

The bean mash reduces the G.I., and the herbs and chile liven up what can be quite a heavy dish. If you prefer to make this in advance and reheat from cold, then allow about 45 minutes in an oven preheated to 425°F.

SERVES 6

1¼ pounds lean lamb, coarsely ground (about 2½ cups)
Ground black pepper
2 onions, finely chopped
2 carrots, chopped
2 stalks of celery, finely sliced
½ teaspoon ground cinnamon
½ teaspoon thyme leaves
½ teaspoon chopped rosemary
¼ cup cornstarch
4 teaspoons tomato paste
2 teaspoons Worcestershire sauce
1¼ cups red wine
1 cup lamb or chicken broth

Bean mash
2 tablespoons extra-virgin olive oil
5 garlic cloves
2 sprigs of fresh rosemary
1 large dried chile
Three x 15-ounce cans of cannellini beans, drained and
    rinsed (if unavailable, use another type of white bean)
About 1¼ cups chicken broth
½ cup coarsely chopped flat-leaf parsley
6 scallions, finely sliced
1 teaspoon very finely chopped rosemary
Ground black pepper

1 Season the lamb with pepper. Heat a large nonstick pan and when hot, add the lamb and brown the meat—it will probably need to be done in batches. You only want to brown the meat, not cook it.

2 Drain each batch of lamb over a bowl and set aside. Once the fat in the bowl has coagulated, reserve 2 teaspoons of it

along with any meat juices. Wipe out the pan and add the 2 teaspoons fat and the vegetables and season with pepper and cinnamon. Then add the chopped herbs. Cook for 8 minutes until the vegetables begin to soften.

3 Add the lamb and cook over medium heat for a few minutes. Add the cornstarch, tomato paste, and Worcestershire sauce. Stir to combine everything thoroughly.

4 Add ½ cup red wine and heat it until its reduced to about 2 tablespoons liquid. Add another ½ cup wine, reduce again, and then add the last ¼ cup and reduce. Pour in the broth, the reserved meat juices, and about 1¼ cups water and bring to a simmer.

5 Cook for about 1 hour. If the sauce becomes too thick during the cooking time, add a little extra water, but remember you don't want the mixture to be too thin. During the last 30 minutes of cooking, make the bean mash.

6 To make the mash, pour the oil into a saucepan over low heat. Add the garlic, rosemary, and chile and cook until the garlic and chile are golden in color. Discard the garlic, rosemary, and chile and keep the oil warm.

7 Meanwhile heat the beans in the chicken broth (you want enough broth just to cover the beans). Cook until the beans are hot but not boiling. Drain, retaining the liquor. Place half the beans in a food processor and blend until smooth. With the machine running, add the warm oil. With a rubber spatula, scrape the puree into a bowl and fold in the whole beans and the remaining ingredients with enough broth to give a spreadable consistency. Season with black pepper to taste.

8 Once the shepherd's pie meat is ready, ladle it into a large ovenproof dish, level out the top, and spoon the bean mash over the top. Finish the pie in a very hot oven (425°F) for 15–20 minutes or under a preheated broiler to become slightly golden.

Per portion: 411 cal., 14g fat, 4.5g sat. fat, 0.41g sodium, 11g carbohydrate

barley "risotto"

Here I used barley instead of arborio rice, which has a high G.I. This also means there is much less stirring!

SERVES: 4–6

2 teaspoons unsalted butter
2 leeks, sliced and rinsed
2 garlic cloves, finely chopped
1/2 teaspoon soft thyme leaves
12 ounces (about 13/4–2 cups) barley or
    brown whole-grain barley
1/2 teaspoon cayenne pepper
About 5 cups chicken broth
4 ounces chorizo sausage, chopped (about 1 cup)
2 handfuls of mixed spinach and arugula
1/4 cup chopped flat-leaf parsley
2 tablespoons chopped chives
1/2 cup freshly grated Parmesan

1 Melt the butter in a large pot over a medium heat. Add the leeks, garlic, and thyme. Cook for 3–4 minutes until the leeks have started to soften, adding a dash of water if necessary to prevent sticking.

2 Stir in the barley, cayenne, and chicken broth. Bring to a boil, reduce the heat, and simmer, covered, until the liquid has evaporated and the barley is tender, adding a little extra broth as necessary—this should take about 40 minutes.

3 Add the chorizo, spinach, and arugula and stir through until the leaves have just wilted.

4 Sprinkle with the herbs and serve topped with the Parmesan.

Per portion: 498 cal., 14g fat, 5.7g sat. fat, 0.71g sodium, 80g carbohydrate

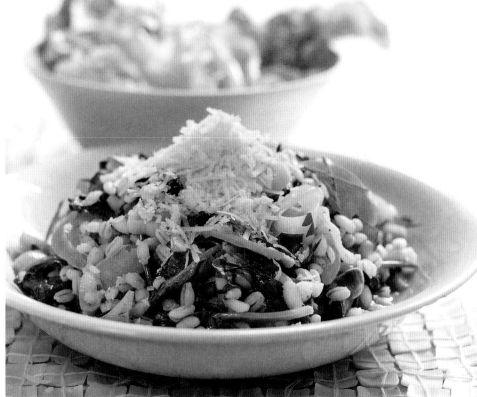

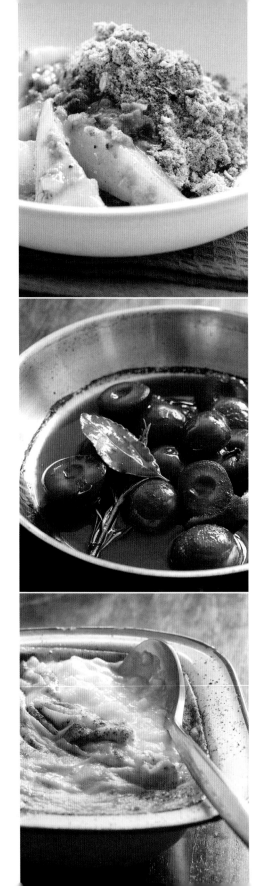

desserts

cherry bread pudding

There are many variations on this bread pudding—try using different fruits.

SERVES 6–8

2^1/$_2$ cups 2% or low-fat milk
1 vanilla bean, split
3 eggs
^{1}/$_4$ cup light brown sugar
6 thick slices whole-grain bread, crusts removed
9 tablespoons cherry spread
2 ounces (about ^{1}/$_3$ cup) dried cherries

1 Bring the milk to a boil with the vanilla bean.

2 Whisk the eggs and sugar and pour in the milk. Scrape the seeds from the vanilla bean into the mixture.

3 Cover the bread with cherry spread and cut in quarters. Arrange in a shallow baking dish and strain the egg and milk mixture over. Sprinkle with the cherries and let soak for about 2 hours.

4 Preheat the oven to 325°F. Cook the pudding in a hot water bath for 25–30 minutes until just set. Serve warm.

Per portion: 383 cal., 7g fat, 2.3g sat. fat, 0.53g sodium, 72g carbohydrate

summer pudding

This is a classic English pudding, using summer berries such as red currants, raspberries, and black currants, but you could use any kind of berry, including blackberries. Save a few berries for decorating the pudding.

SERVES 8

2 pounds raspberries (about 6 cups)
8 ounces (about 2 cups) red currants, picked over
2 ounces (about ^{1}/$_2$ cup) black currants, picked over
^{1}/$_2$ cup light brown sugar
10–12 slices of day-old whole-grain bread, crusts removed
^{1}/$_2$ cup cherry brandy
Extra berries, for decorating

1 Sprinkle the fruit with the sugar and toss gently to combine. Cover and let it macerate for 2 hours.

2 Meanwhile, line a 4-pint pudding bowl with plastic wrap then with slices of bread. Make sure the bread overlaps slightly and covers the sides and bottom completely.

3 Tip the fruit and resulting juices into a nonreactive saucepan along with the cherry brandy and cook over medium heat for 3–4 minutes to release some more juices.

4 Using a slotted spoon, fill up the bread mold with the fruit. Pour in half the juices, then cover the fruit completely with more bread slices. Cover with plastic wrap, then top with a plate that fits into the rim of the bowl. Place a heavy weight on top of the plate and refrigerate overnight.

5 When ready to serve, turn the bowl over onto a shallow, but not flat dish and remove the bowl and plastic wrap. Pour the reserved juices over it and serve with a few loose berries.

Per portion: 263 cal., 2g fat, 0.4g sat. fat, 0.32g sodium, 52g carbohydrate

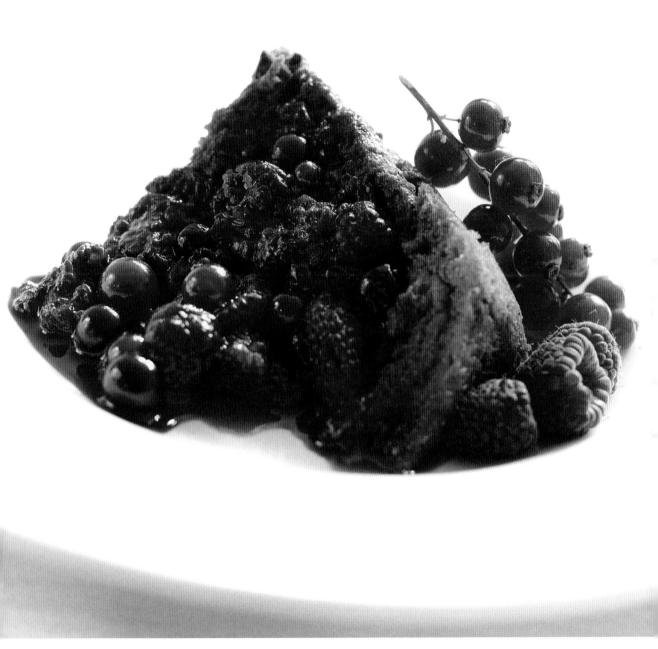

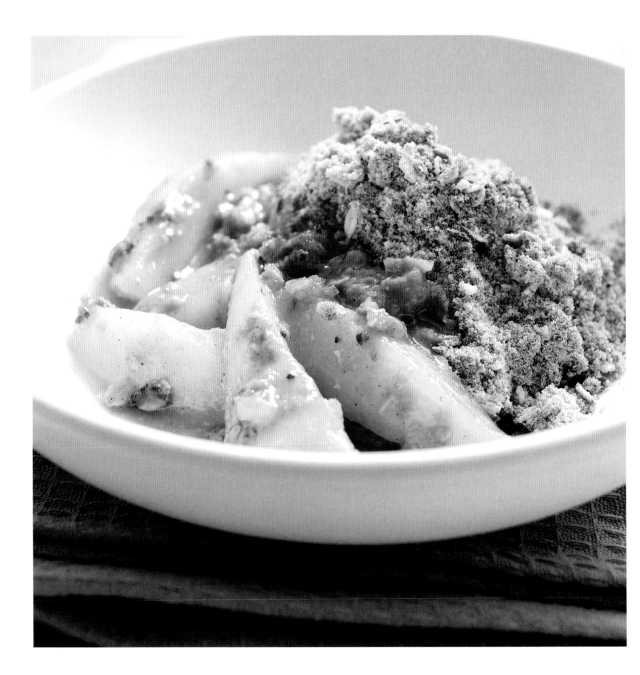

pear crumble

This has a very fine textured topping which absorbs the delicious juices from the pears, citrus zest, and nutmeg.

SERVES 6–8

8 ripe Bosc pears, peeled, cored, and sliced
Finely grated zest of 1 orange and 1 lemon
2 tablespoons light brown sugar
Pinch of grated nutmeg
5 tablespoons reduced-fat powdered milk
$1/4$ cup ground almonds
$1/2$ cup rolled oats
$1^1/3$ cups whole-grain flour
$1/2$ cup soft dark brown sugar
1 teaspoon ground cinnamon
3 tablespoons unsalted butter, softened

1 Preheat the oven to 400°F.

2 Combine the pears with the zest, sugar, nutmeg, and $1/2$ cup water in the bottom of a large baking dish.

3 Mix the dry ingredients together, then rub in the butter.

4 Sprinkle this mixture on top of the pears and bake for 45 minutes to 1 hour, or until the top is golden. Serve warm with low-sugar custard.

Per portion (excluding custard): 433 cal., 10g fat, 3.8g sat. fat, 0.04g sodium, 85g carbohydrate

drunken berries

Macerating fruit in alcohol and sugar softens them and fills them with lovely flavors. Berries have a low G.I. and are packed full of vitamins, so this is an easy, virtually fat-free way to enjoy them.

SERVES 4–6

8-ounce carton strawberries (about 2 cups),
*   hulled and quartered*
6-ounce carton raspberries, (about $1^1/4$ cups), picked over
5-ounce carton blackberries (about $1^1/4$ cups), picked over
5-ounce carton red currants (about $1^1/3$–$1^1/2$ cups),
*   berries removed from their stems*
$1/4$ cup crème de cassis (black currant liqueur)
1 tablespoon confectioners' sugar
1 tablespoon lemon juice (optional)

1 In a glass bowl, combine all the fruits gently with the cassis, confectioners' sugar, and lemon juice, if using. Let them macerate for about 3 hours, turning the fruits from time to time.

2 Serve on their own or with low-fat plain yogurt.

Per portion: 124 cal, 0.3g fat, 0.0g sat. fat, 0.01g sodium, 23g carbohydrate

whole poached apricots

Typically Mediterranean, this is also incredibly easy to make. To remove the pits from fresh apricots, just make a small cut and the pit will come out easily—don't cut the apricots all the way through. If you can't find fresh apricots, you could use dried apricots, but cut the amount in half and soak for several hours in cold water until plump.

SERVES 6

1/3 cup light brown sugar
4 green cardamom pods, crushed
2 teaspoons fresh lemon juice
2 1/4 pounds ripe apricots (about 6–7 cups), split, pit removed
   (or around 20–25 dried apricots, reconstituted)
2 ounces slivered almonds or pine nuts (about 1/2 cup), toasted
Pomegranate seeds (optional)

1 Preheat the oven to 350°F.

2 Pour 2 1/2 cups water into a wide flameproof and ovenproof pan with the sugar, cardamom, and lemon juice and bring to a boil. When boiling, add the apricots and remove from the heat. Cover them with wet parchment paper, put the lid on the pan and place in the oven. Cook for 20–30 minutes. Remove from the oven and let cool in the syrup.

3 To serve, remove the apricots and drain, reserving the syrup. Top with the slivered toasted almonds and pomegranate seeds, if using, and pour some of the syrup over them.

Per portion: 153 cal., 5g fat, 0.4g sat. fat, 0.01g sodium, 26g carbohydrate

compote of plums in spiced rosemary syrup

This is luscious. Very like mulled wine, but with plums, all the flavors intensify and combine to make a lovely thick syrup.

SERVES 4

2/3 cup red wine
1/4 cup sugar
Sprig of rosemary
1 bay leaf
1 strip each lemon and orange zest
2 whole cloves
2-inch piece of cinnamon stick
18 ounces red plums, cut in half and pitted (about 2 1/2–3 cups)

1 Bring the first seven ingredients to a boil and simmer until the sugar has dissolved. Add the plums and cover with a lid. Cook gently until the plums are just tender.

2 Remove the plums and set aside. If you like, boil the juices to reduce slightly. Pour the juices over the plums and serve warm or cold with low-fat plain yogurt.

Per portion: 125 cal., 0.2g fat, 0.0g sat. fat, 0.01g sodium, 25g carbohydrate

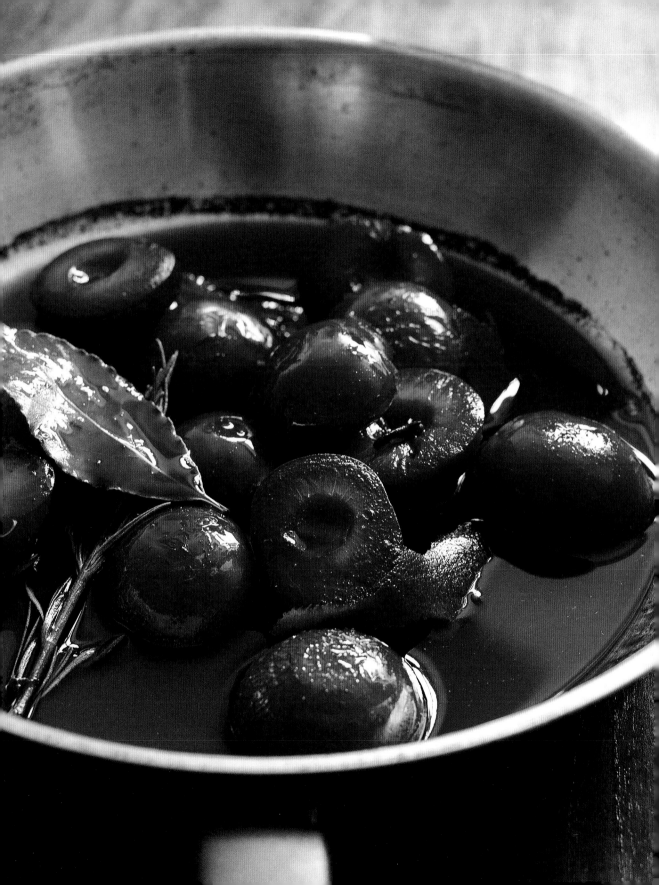

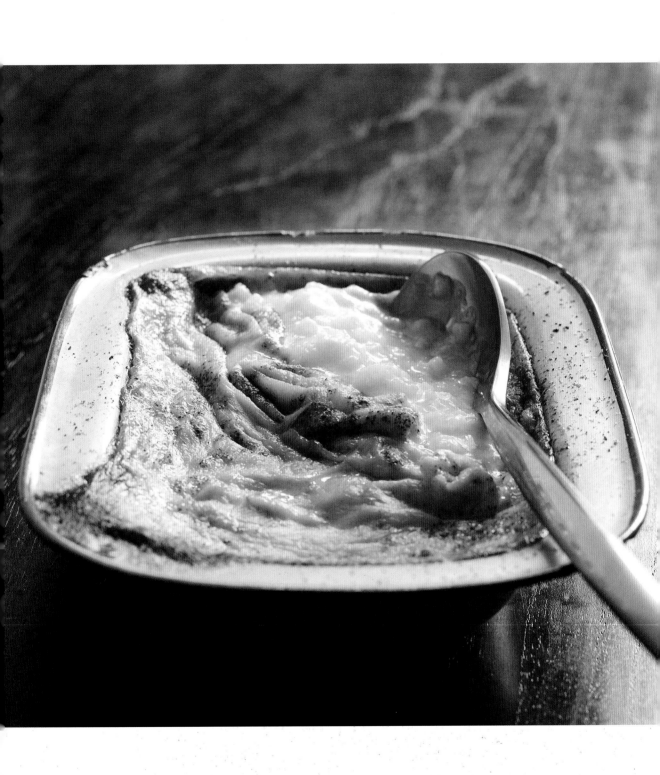

rice pudding

Rice puddings have to be cooked slowly for best results, but it is comfort food for all the family. If you are using brown short-grain rice, cover it with cold water and bring to a boil. Reduce the heat and simmer for 15 minutes, then drain and continue as below. You will also need more rice—²⁄₃ cup—and to cook it for longer—2–3 hours.

SERVES 4–6

6 ¹⁄₂ cups short-grain rice
Pinch of salt
¹⁄₄ cup light brown sugar
4–5 cups skim milk
Grated nutmeg or cinnamon
2 tablespoons butter

1 Preheat the oven to 300°F.

2 Wash and drain the rice and put in a 1¹⁄₂–2 quart baking dish.

3 Add a pinch of salt, the sugar, and 4 cups milk, and stir. Sprinkle grated nutmeg or cinnamon over it and top with pats of butter. Bake in the center or towards the bottom of the oven for about 2 hours. Stir in the skin that forms on the top at least once during the cooking time, adding extra milk as necessary.

Per portion: 235 cal., 6g fat, 3.9g sat. fat, 0.25g sodium, 39g carbohydrate

baked peaches

Peaches are just as good cooked as they are fresh. This is a really simple recipe, but it looks wonderful when it comes out of the oven.

SERVES 4

Juice of 1 lime
Pinch of grated nutmeg
2 tablespoons soft brown sugar
2 tablespoons unsalted butter, softened
¹⁄₄ cup chopped toasted hazelnuts
4 ripe peaches (yellow or white), cut in half and pit removed

1 Preheat the oven to 375°F.

2 Mix together the lime juice, nutmeg, sugar, butter, and hazelnuts.

3 Place the peaches, cut side up, in a baking dish in which they fit snugly, and divide the sugar mixture between the peach halves. Bake for about 20 minutes until the syrup is bubbling and there are golden-brown flecks on the peaches. Baste the peaches occasionally with the syrupy juices that come from them while they are cooking. Serve warm.

Per portion: 160 cal., 9g fat, 3.6g sat. fat, 0.01g sodium, 19g carbohydrate

baked apples with fruit and nuts

Small British Bramley apples are perfect for this dish as they cook to a soft puree encased in lightly caramelized skins. Large dessert apples could also be used.

SERVES 4

4 small cooking apples, each weighing about 8 ounces
2 tablespoons soft dark brown sugar
4 tablespoons sweet mincemeat
1/4 cup slivered almonds or chopped pecans
1 teaspoon ground cinnamon
Butter, for greasing
About 2/3 cup apple juice for basting

1 Preheat the oven to 375°F.

2 Remove the center core from the apples, leaving 1/4-inch uncut at the bottom. Run the tip of a sharp knife around the circumference of the apple, just to pierce the skin—this will stop the apples bursting in the oven.

3 Combine the remaining ingredients except the juice and press into the cavities of the apples. Place them in a buttered baking dish in which they fit snugly, then pour in 2 tablespoons apple juice and pop in the oven for 45 minutes to 1 hour. At 10-minute intervals, add 2 more tablespoons apple juice to the bottom of the dish and spoon the juices over the apples. Serve warm.

Per portion: 251 cal., 5g fat, 0.3g sat. fat, 0.02g sodium, 53g carbohydrate

herby fruit salad

A twist on a classic fruit salad, the Asian influence of cilantro and coconut milk is unusual yet refreshing—perfect after a heavy meal.

SERVES 4–6

1/4 cup reduced-fat coconut milk
1 tablespoon honey
Lemon or lime juice, to taste
2 blood oranges or small pink grapefruit, peeled and sliced
1 small pineapple, peeled and chopped
1 pink-skinned apple, cored and chopped
1 banana, peeled and sliced
1 small mango, peeled and chopped
2 tablespoons chopped cilantro

Mix the coconut milk, honey, and lemon juice. Toss the fruits and cilantro in this dressing.

Per portion: 141 cal., 0.5g fat, 0.1g sat. fat, 0.02g sodium, 34g carbohydrate

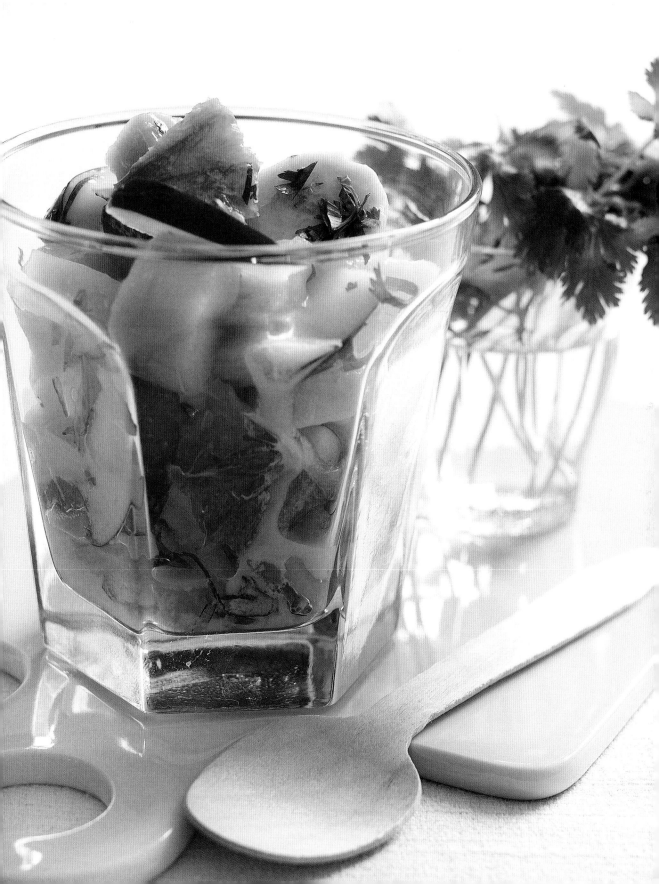

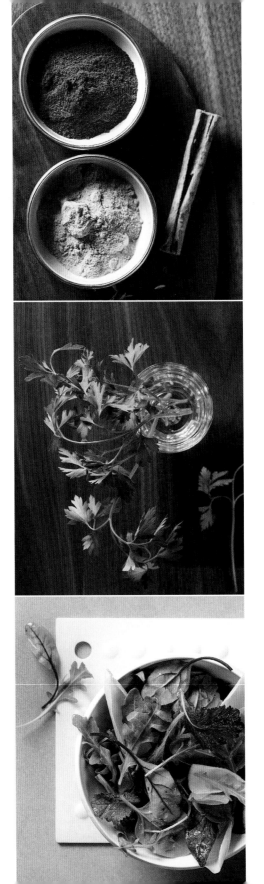

sauces and accompaniments

rich tomato sauce

This is an excellent recipe that can be used as a base for many dishes. Or serve it with gnocchi or whole-wheat pasta.

SERVES 6–8—MAKES ABOUT 1 QUART

1 tablespoon extra-virgin olive oil
1 onion, finely chopped
2 garlic cloves, finely chopped
1 stick of celery, finely chopped
2/3 cup dry white wine
1 pound, 10 ounces plum tomatoes, peeled, seeded and
    chopped (about 3 cups), or Two x 14 1/2-ounce cans of
    chopped tomatoes
1 fresh bay leaf
1 teaspoon tomato paste
Handful of roughly chopped fresh herbs, such as flat-leaf
    parsley, marjoram, and basil
Ground black pepper

1 Heat a heavy pot and add the olive oil, then stir in the onion, garlic, and celery, and cook for about 5 minutes until softened but not colored, stirring occasionally. Pour in the wine and let it bubble away, then add the tomatoes along with the bay leaf and tomato paste.

2 Bring the sauce to a boil, then simmer gently, uncovered, for about 30 minutes, stirring occasionally until the sauce is well reduced and thickened. Remove from the heat and let cool a little.

3 When the sauce has cooled, remove the bay leaf and stir in the herbs. Season to taste with black pepper and reheat gently to use as needed.

Per 1/3 cup: 36 cal., 1g fat, 0.2g sat. fat, 0.01g sodium, 7g carbohydrate

parsley sauce

A classic British recipe that is great with fish or vegetables.

SERVES 4—MAKES 1 1/4 CUPS

2 teaspoons unsalted butter
2 tablespoons cornstarch
1 1/2–2 cups skim milk
3 tablespoons chopped fresh parsley
Handful of fresh sorrel leaves, shredded (optional)
Ground white pepper

1 Melt the butter in a small pan. Add the cornstarch, stirring. Pour in the milk, a little at a time, beating vigorously until smooth after each addition. Simmer gently for 2–3 minutes until smooth and thickened, stirring occasionally.

2 Add the parsley and sorrel, if using, and reheat gently until the sorrel has just wilted. Season with white pepper to taste.

Per 1/3 cup: 72 cal., 2g fat, 1.2g sat. fat, 0.04g sodium, 14g carbohydrate

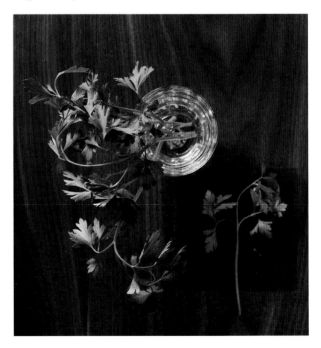

red onion marmalade

Tasty with cheese or cold meats, spread a little onto a crostini before topping with other ingredients. If you like, you can use white onions, white wine, and white wine vinegar, but add raisins instead of prunes. This makes a great gift.

SERVES 10—MAKES 2¼ cups

2 tablespoons unsalted butter
1 pound, 10 ounces red onions, thinly sliced (around 6½–7 cups)
½ teaspoon coarse salt (e.g., Kosher salt)
1 bay leaf
1 teaspoon fresh thyme leaves
½ teaspoon ground black pepper
¼ cup light brown sugar
1 tablespoon dry sherry
1 tablespoon aged red wine vinegar
Scant cup red wine
1 tablespoon honey
2 ounces pitted prunes (about ⅓–½ cup), chopped

1 Melt the butter in a heavy pot over medium heat. Add the onions, salt, bay leaf, thyme, and pepper. Stir to combine. Reduce the heat, cover, and cook for about 30 minutes, stirring from time to time, and adding a splash of water if it starts to stick.

2 Remove the lid and add the remaining ingredients. Cook over a very low heat until it becomes dark in color, about 45 minutes. Keep a look out for burning towards the end of cooking. Stir regularly.

3 Cool and store in sterilized glass jars, refrigerated. This will keep for 2 months.

Per ⅓ cup: 83 cal., 2g fat, 1.2g sat. fat, 0.09g sodium, 15g carbohydrate

cilantro mint chutney

Delicious as chutney, this also makes a great dip if you fold it into low-fat plain yogurt. Eat with poppadoms and tandoori dishes.

MAKES ⅔ CUP

1 ounce mint leaves (about 2 handfuls)
1½ ounces cilantro leaves (about 2½–3 cups)
½ small onion, roughly chopped
½-inch piece fresh ginger, peeled and chopped
½ chile, seeded and roughly chopped
¼ teaspoon cumin seeds
1 small garlic clove
½ teaspoon salt
½ tablespoon lemon juice
½ tablespoon dry, unsweetened coconut, moistened in ½ tablespoon water

Blend all the ingredients in a food processor until well combined. It will keep for a few days if you store in an airtight container in the refrigerator.

Per ⅓ cup: 73 cal., 5g fat, 3.8g sat. fat, 0.56g sodium, 8g carbohydrate

pickled blackberries

A pickle relish that goes well with cheese or cold meats such as duck. Blackberries are also a superfruit as they contain so much goodness—the antioxidant vitamins C and E as well as fiber. They also have a lovely rich color.

SERVES 10

18 ounces blackberries (about 3^1/$_2$–4 cups)
1^1/$_4$ cups light brown sugar
1 teaspoon ground allspice
1 tablespoon ground ginger
^{2}/$_3$ cup white wine vinegar

1 In a bowl, combine the blackberries, sugar, and spices, stir through, cover, and let marinate overnight.

2 Bring the vinegar to a boil, add the berries, and simmer gently, uncovered, for 20 minutes.

3 Let cool and spoon into sterilized jars. This will keep for a couple of months in the fridge.

Per ^{1}/$_3$ cup: 118 cal., 0.1g fat, 0.0g sat. fat, 0.01g sodium, 28g carbohydrate

sweet pickled onions

The best pickling recipe I have tried, especially if you like your onions a little sweet. Salting is the first stage of this recipe, and although a large amount of salt is used here, a lot of it is discarded before pickling. Be warned, this needs to be made over a couple of days.

MAKES TWO LARGE JARS (ABOUT 1 QUART)

2^1/$_2$ pounds peeled pearl onions or baby onions
   (about 9^1/$_2$–10^1/$_2$ cups)
3 tablespoons salt
^{1}/$_2$ cup soft brown sugar
^{1}/$_3$ cup golden syrup (if unavailable, use corn syrup)
1 teaspoon whole cloves
1 tablespoon black peppercorns
2 red chiles, quartered and seeded
Pinch of mustard seeds
2-inch piece of cinnamon stick
1 bay leaf
Sprig of thyme
3 slices ginger
2^1/$_2$ cups malt vinegar (if unavailable, use apple cider vinegar)

1 Mix the onions with the salt and leave overnight.

2 In a nonreactive saucepan, combine the sugar, golden syrup, cloves, peppercorns, chiles, mustard seeds, cinnamon, bay leaf, thyme, ginger, and malt vinegar. Bring to a boil, remove from the heat, and let cool overnight.

3 The next day, drain and dry the onions and pack into sterilized storage jars. Boil the pickling liquor and pour it over the onions, evenly distributing the herbs and spices.

4 Seal the jars and store for 2 weeks before eating. Once opened, they will keep for several months in the fridge.

Per ^{1}/$_3$ cup: 54 cal., 0.1g fat, 0.0g sat. fat, 1.00g sodium, 12g carbohydrate

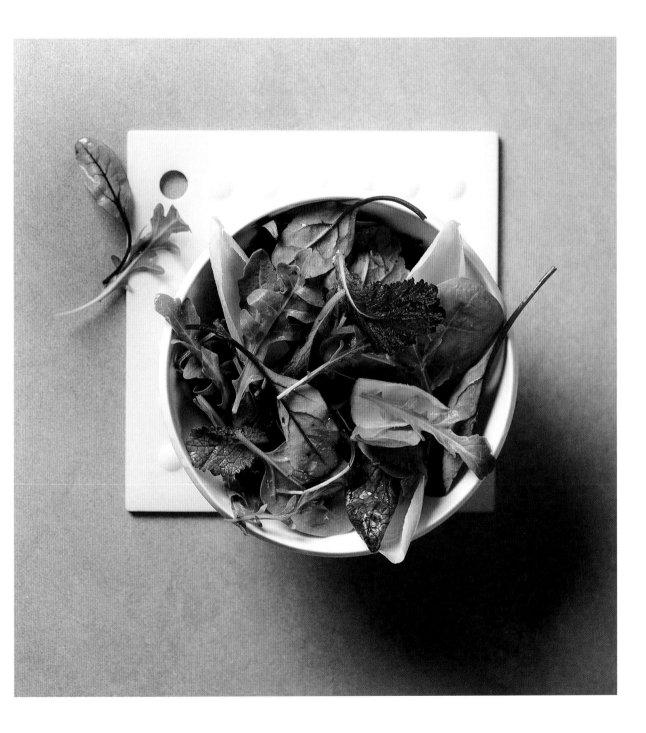

Index

acknowledgments

There are too many people to thank but certain individuals deserve a special mention:

To my wonderful wife, Jacinta, and our two children, Toby and Billie, who suffered from my lack of quality time yet supported me throughout as I managed to juggle my time through two books and everything else going on in my life.

To Louise, my energetic and ultra-efficient personal assistant, who fielded hundreds of phone calls from the publishers and who was regularly on hand to smooth troubled waters when the pressures of deadlines occasionally took their toll.

To Fiona Lindsay, Linda Shanks, and Lesley Turnbull at Limelight Management who are constantly there to make sure I have more than enough work to handle.

To my team at Notting Grill and Kew Grill, especially David, George, Antonio, and Candido, who kept the boat afloat in my often extended absences.

To the various friends Nicki, Kate, Sarah, John and Anne, June, Mike, and Nicky who acted unknowingly as guinea pigs for many of the recipes.

To Dr. Mabel Blades for her guidance on the G.I. and Jane Suthering for her creativity in helping to make my recipes G.I.-friendly.

And finally to Muna Reyal, my editor and her fab team at Kyle Cathie, for giving me the opportunity to produce this cookbook. They turned my offerings into a beautifully executed book.
—Antony Worrall Thompson

I would like to thank my husband, Peter Blades, for his love and encouragement as well as for helping me to keep the midnight oil burning. And thanks also to Daisy Rose, my long-time Australian friend for her great interest and support.

I have also really enjoyed working with Antony and Jane, especially as we all spoke the same language about food, and I would like to thank my editor, Muna, for holding my hand throughout and giving us cakes and wine in the office.
—Mabel Blades

As ever, creating a book is all about team work—and what a great team it's been. We've prepared and tasted every recipe—as many as 7 in a day sometimes—and even so I've still managed to lose a few pounds in weight. I'm certainly a G.I. convert!
—Jane Suthering

bibliography

Nutrition and Health
by Mabel Blades
Highfield Books

The New Glucose Revolution
by Anthony Leeds, Jennie Brand-Miller, Kaye Foster-Powell, and Stephen Colagiuri
Hodder Mobius

The G.I. Point Diet
by Azmina Govindji and Nina Puddefoot
Vermilion

Healthy Eating for Diabetes
by Antony Worrall Thompson and Azmina Govindji
Kyle Cathie Ltd.

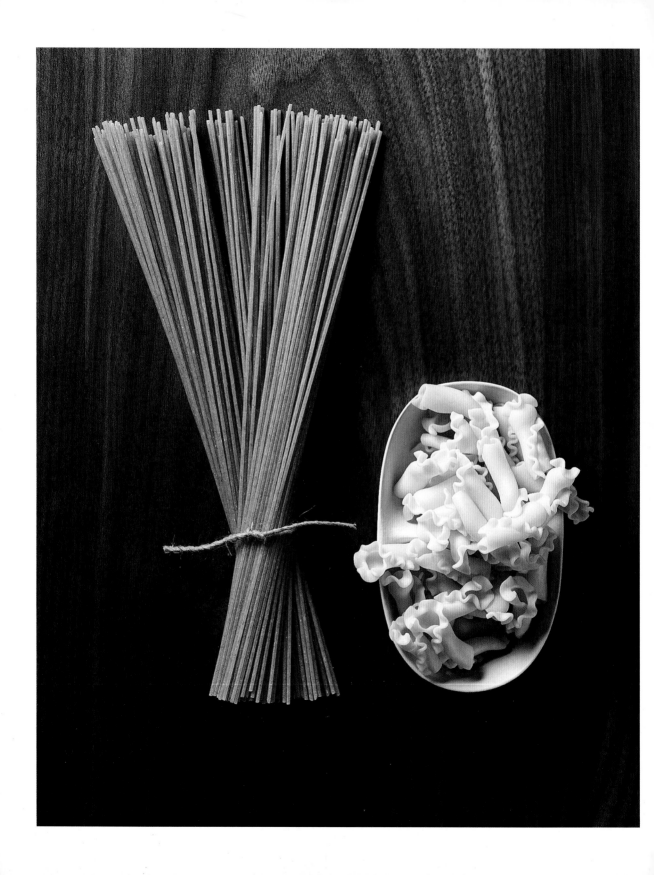

the g̅.i̲. diet cookbook

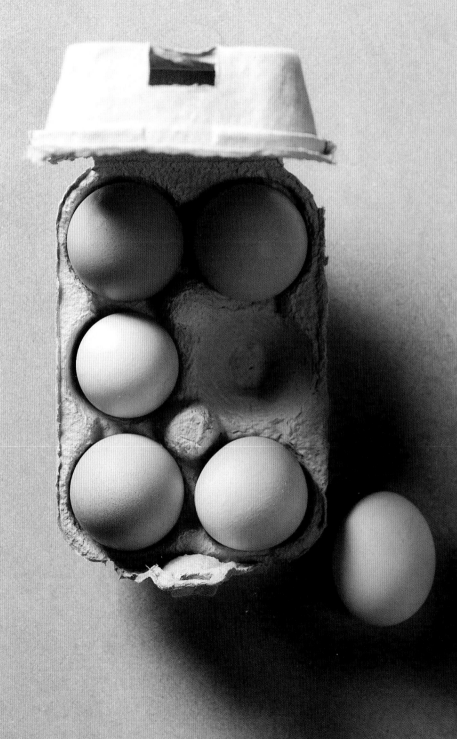

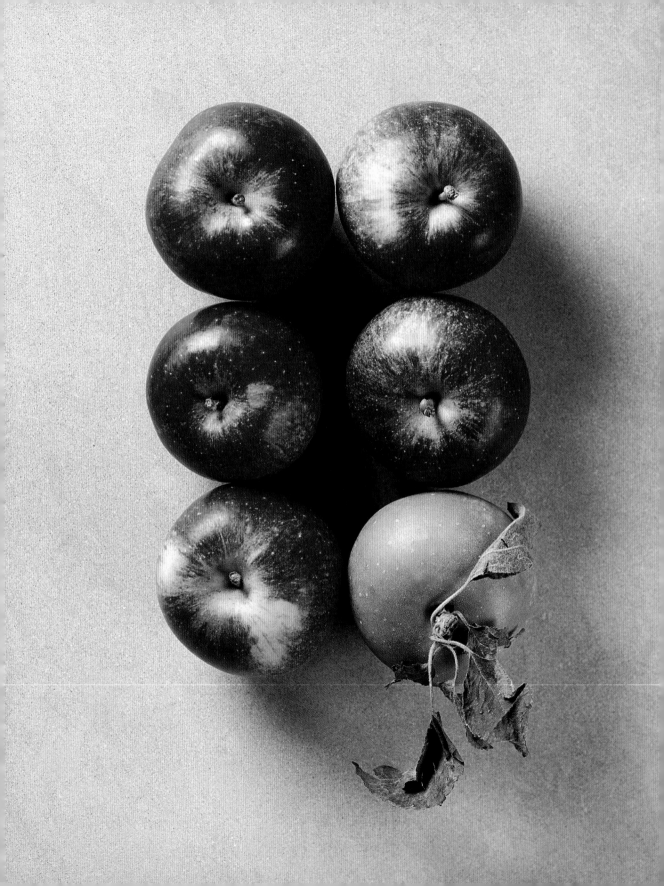